# Conservative Dentistry
An integrated approach

CHURCHILL LIVINGSTONE DENTAL SERIES

**A Manual of Paedodontics**
Second edition
*R. J. Andlaw and W. P Rock*

**Clinical Pharmacology in Dentistry**
Fifth edition
*R. A. Cawson and R. G. Spector*

**Essentials of Dental Surgery and Pathology**
Fourth edition
*R. A. Cawson*

**Notes on Dental Materials**
Fifth edition
*E. C. Combe*

**Anatomy for Students of Dentistry**
Fifth edition
*A. D. Dixon*

**An Introduction to Removable Denture Prosthetics**
*A. A. Grant and W. Johnson*

**Occlusion in Restorative Dentistry**
Technique and theory
*M. D. Gross and J. Dewe-Mathews*

**Essentials of Pathology for Dental Students**
*W. Lawler, A. Ahmed and W. J. Hulme*

**Clinical Anatomy for Dentistry**
*R. B. Longmore and D. A. McRae*

**Dental and Maxillofacial Radiology**
*J. McIvor*

**Principles and Practice of Orthodontics**
Second edition
*J. R. E. Mills*

**Introduction to Dental Anatomy**
Ninth edition
*J. H. Scott and N. B. B. Symons*

**Principles of Pathology for Dental Students**
Fourth edition
*J. B. Walter, M. C. Hamilton and M. S. Israel*

**Basic and Applied Dental Biochemistry**
Second edition
*R. A. D. Williams and J. C. Elliott*

# Conservative Dentistry
## An integrated approach

Edited by

**P. H. Jacobsen** MDS (Lond) FDSRCS (Eng)
Senior Lecturer in Conservative Dentistry,
University of Wales College of Medicine,
Cardiff;
Honorary Consultant Dental Surgeon,
South Glamorgan Health Authority, UK

CHURCHILL LIVINGSTONE
EDINBURGH LONDON MELBOURNE AND NEW YORK 1990

CHURCHILL LIVINGSTONE
Medical Division of Longman Group UK Limited

Distributed in the United States of America by
Churchill Livingstone Inc., 1560 Broadway, New York,
N.Y. 10036, and by associated companies, branches
and representatives throughout the world.

First published 1990

ISBN 0-443-03958-5

**British Library Cataloguing in Publication Data**
Conservative dentistry.
    1. Conservative dentistry
    I. Jacobsen, P. H.
    617.6'01

**Library of Congress Cataloging in Publication Data**
Conservative dentistry: an integrated approach/edited by P. H.
Jacobsen
        p.      cm.
    Bibliography: p.
    ISBN 0-443-03958-5
    1. Fillings (Dentistry)  2. Dental caries — Treatment.  3. Dental
pulp — Diseases — Treatment.  I. Jacobsen, P. H. (Peter H.)
    [DNLM: 1. Dental Caries — therapy.  2. Dental Pulp Diseases —
therapy.  3. Dental Restoration, Permanent.  WU 270 C755]
    RK517.C66  1990
    617.6'7 — dc20
    DNLM/DLC                                89-15869
    for Library of Congress                     CIP

Produced by Longman Singapore Publishers (Pte) Ltd.
Printed in Singapore

# Preface

The senior undergraduate and newly qualified practitioner are not well served by practical textbooks in conservative dentistry which discuss clinical techniques and materials in the context of the limitations imposed by the patient, and the ability and facilities of the dentist.

Technique manuals and laboratory benchbooks are excellent in their scope, and large reference books give encyclopaedic detail of operative techniques. However, the constraints of the patient and the environment of the restoration impose restrictions on the choice and execution of techniques.

The middle ground, of techniques matched to the patient and the skill of the operator, is hardly occupied, and this book stakes a claim for it.

In addition, many elementary books do not give authorative views on the relationship of oral biology and pathology, dental materials science and dental technology to the clinical techniques of conservative dentistry. This book draws on the specialist experience of its authors in these fields.

Whilst the authors agree with the continuing trend to integrate the three clinical restorative subjects, they believe that conservative dentistry with its intimate relationships with the tooth, saliva, materials and, not least, the patient, is still deserving of its own textbooks.

This book is not intended to be a technique manual, nor an encyclopaedic reference book; it is more in the style of seminar discussions which would be equally at home in senior undergraduate teaching, vocational training or with junior hospital staff. It assumes that a basic level of knowledge has already been acquired from technique courses and seeks to build on this. Some chapters are intended to revise and organize earlier learning and others are written to introduce more demanding subjects from a basic and practical viewpoint. There will always be a need to read extensive texts, and a bibliography has been compiled to guide further reading.

The authors believe that undergraduates, in particular, have difficulty in organizing information into a logical sequence for decision making. Flow charts have been included to help overcome this problem and to show that no matter how complex a subject is, there is always a step-wise series of decisions involved, each decision inevitably excluding many other options. The undergraduate tends to present all the options (when he or she knows them), rather than being selective and discarding early on those which are not applicable to that particular patient.

We have tried to eliminate the small print and concentrate on percentage dentistry — the type of dentistry that bring success most often, for the satisfaction of both the dentist and the patient.

Cardiff, 1989 P. H. J.

*To Charlotte:*
*for whom learning is one of the greatest*
*pleasures of life.*

# Acknowledgements

Many people have helped in the gestation and production of this book.

Professor Richard Johns was involved in the early discussions about the form of the book, and we thank him for his enthusiasm and encouragement.

Several friends have been very helpful — Professor Michael Braden, Dr Peter Staheli and Dr Alan Atkinson have read and criticized chapters and have given moral support; sincere thanks to them.

Mr Frank Hartles and the staff of the Audiovisual Aids Department at Cardiff have contributed greatly through the clinical photographs and much of the artwork — in particular Mr Ron Lambert, Mr Rodney Doller and Mrs Jo Griffiths all deserve a personal mention and thanks. The remainder of the artwork was done by Mr Peter Cox, freelance medical artist, and we thank him for his efforts.

Mr Jeff Lock and Mr Reg Day constructed much of the (successful!) technical work shown in the book, and thanks are due to them for their skills and for continuing the essential partnership of technician and clinician. Whilst drawing attention to teamwork, thanks are due to Miss Sally King, dental surgery assistant, for participating in the chairside work for these cases.

The staff of Churchill Livingstone, particularly Mr Simon Fathers and Miss Máire Collins, have provided help and encouragement in the production of the book — we thank them sincerely.

Mrs Karen Jacobsen typed much of the manuscript, but more importantly, tolerated the many hours of editing which deprived her of her husband from domestic duties — we're glad it's over!!

Finally, all our undergraduates and postgraduates provided the inspiration to put this together — we hope they like it!

P. H. J.

# Contributors

**Peter H. Jacobsen** MDS(Lond) FDSRCS(Eng)
Senior Lecturer in Conservative Dentistry,
University of Wales College of Medicine, Cardiff;
Honorary Consultant Dental Surgeon, South
Glamorgan Health Authority, UK

**David K. Whittaker** PhD(Wales) BDS(Manc)
FDSRCS(Eng)
Reader in Oral Biology, University of Wales
College of Medicine, Cardiff; Honorary
Consultant Dental Surgeon, South Glamorgan
Health Authority, UK

**John D. Lilley** PhD MSc LDS(Manc) FDSRCPS(Glas)
Senior Lecturer in Conservative Dentistry,
Turner Dental School, University of
Manchester; Honorary Consultant in Restorative
Dentistry, Manchester Health Authority, UK

**Gavin J. Pearson** PhD BDS(Lond) LDSRCS(Eng)
Senior Lecturer in Conservative Dentistry,
University College, London, Dental School;
Honorary Consultant Dental Surgeon,
Bloomsbury District Health Authority, UK

**Robin Huggett** MSc(Bath) CGIA FTC
Lecturer and Chief Instructor, University of
Bristol Dental School, Bristol, UK

**Richard J. Garn** FTC LCG
Instructor, Department of Conservative
Dentistry, University of Bristol Dental School,
Bristol, UK

# Contents

# The patient

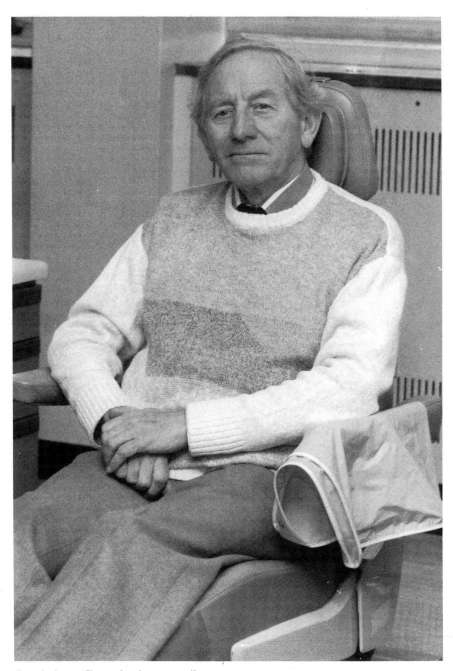

**Frontispiece** 'I'm ready when you are!'

# 1. The patient's limitations and expectations

*P. H. Jacobsen   G. J. Pearson*

Many texts on conservative dentistry begin immediately with technical considerations, such as rotary instruments or cavity preparation, or with pathological considerations, such as caries or periodontal disease. This book begins with the most important consideration of all, the real purpose for which *all* the books are written — the patient.

It is usually by the patient's own volition that he seeks conservative advice and treatment, and he usually brings with him certain problems and limitations which influence treatment planning and the delivery of care.

Each patient also attends with strong preconceptions based on their previous experience of dentistry. This could be good or bad; with a single traumatic episode being able to reverse many years of co-operation. The patient will have some idea of what dentistry could or might do for him, and what he wants from his dentist. Some of his concepts could well be limited or unambitious, and education has a major role to play here. Conversely, sometimes his concepts could be over-ambitious, complex bridgework for instance, and here re-education is often necessary to bring him down to the practical and feasible.

It might be that the dentist has the skills and technical facilities to perform advanced procedures, but before bur is put to tooth, the dentist must stop and ask whether this is really what *this* patient needs and wants. If the answer is no, then to proceed is an act of pure selfishness which might also be regarded as negligent.

Certainly the dentist may have certain treatment goals for all his patients — for instance, no pain or caries, healthy periodontium, complete occlusion — but the way in which care is prescribed and delivered has to be tempered by the patient's aspirations for his own mouth and his readiness to accept care.

A prolonged treatment plan could be very inconvenient to a shift worker, or to a mother with young children, or those with no personal transport. It might create restorations which would be beyond the maintenance capacity of the lazy or disinterested, or those with inadequate washing facilities.

Perhaps the patient is a reluctant attender, extremely apprehensive of dental care and its possible discomforts, and will require some form of therapeutic help just to get the simple things done. The short, unambitious treatment plan is more likely to succeed here, and if the patient's confidence can be obtained, the more complex treatment could be provided later.

Advanced restorations require skill and facilities, and these have to be paid for, either by the State or by the patient. Both have limited resources and both deserve value for money. Committing resources to an ambitious treatment plan should involve judgement on the likely lifespan of the restorations in that particular mouth and its conditions, and whether the expense is justifiable.

The intra-oral conditions bring as much influence to bear: the caries rate, the number of missing teeth, the periodontal condition, the presence of dentures and the quality of previous restorative work all act as limitations to the scope of the treatment plan. All of us like to provide our best work for those who will appreciate it and look after it. Disinterest on the dentist's part is created by the appearance of large plaque deposits and evidence of little care.

The other side of the equation is what level of resources is available, which relates to the dentist's skills and training, the available materials and techniques, and the facilities available for providing care (Fig. 1.1). These, in turn, could well modify or

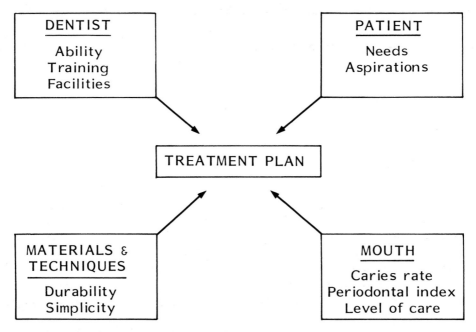

**Fig. 1.1**   Influences on the formulation of a treatment plan.

even dictate the patient's aspirations; a clean, well equipped and efficient practice would indicate a good level of care to the average patient, whilst the reverse could well lower his expectations.

Dentists should offer only what is realistically available and work within their own limitations. It is certainly no disgrace to say that certain options are beyond your capabilities and it is possible to consider referral. It could also be that the options the patient has aspirations towards are those with a lower success rate, and it is sensible to tell him this frankly.

There is considerably greater awareness today of the cosmetic possibilities of modern dentistry, and thus demand for new materials and techniques. Much of this is expensive and has not been fully evaluated over a sufficient period for total confidence in its durability. The patient deserves a proper explanation of the reservations there are about particular lines of treatment.

The provision of restorative treatment is a complex arrangement wherein the patient, the dentist, the technical support and the materials must be in harmony to produce a satisfactory result. The limitations of one element will inevitably change the effects of the others. It is important to remember that the treatment is only as good as its weakest link — don't let that be you!

The key to success throughout is *communication*: listen and learn from what the patient says, explain what *can* be done, and then decide jointly on what *should* be done. If you are not sure, do not commit yourself, but delay the decision and take advice from your colleagues or even your local consultant.

This book begins by discussing how to find out what is wrong with the patient and what *he* wants done about it, coupled with the limitations the patient brings to formulating a treatment plan and then to executing it.

# 2. History and examination

*J. D. Lilley*

The history should provide a clear account of the patient's experience of health care prior to the current attendance. It should establish an organized body of knowledge about the patient's dental past and their fitness to receive future treatment — it forms part of the rationale for their management. The history, though, is very subjective and prone to differences in the perceptions and aspirations of the patient and the dentist. These differences may be reduced or exaggerated by the level of communication between the two, and the dentist must bear this problem in mind.

Clearly, it is the dentist's responsibility to create the right atmosphere for the patient to tell his story. The patient must be sitting comfortably in quiet surroundings and be confident in the dentist's sympathetic attention. He should be sitting upright, not supine and vulnerable, and facing the questioner with his eyes at the same level. This avoids the 'operating' position, with its overtones of discomfort and interrogation.

The most limiting aspect of the history is that to a certain extent it is not strictly factual. It is the patient's *perception* of events or circumstances. Even items of medical history can be incorrectly remembered or misunderstood, and in difficult cases the patient's medical practitioner must be contacted for information. The dental aspects are often muddled, particularly in the identification of a troublesome tooth amongst thirty or so others.

The dentist has to sift this information and organize it, give it the weight it deserves, and then record it and draw conclusions from it. A systematic approach should be used, so as to pick up inconsistencies in the story and not miss anything. However, the dentist must beware of the too precise patient with an obsessively detailed history, which can be just as misleading or unhelpful as that provided by the vague patient. The history should be taken slowly, with pauses for writing in the notes; this helps the patient relax and lets further information come to his mind.

## EVALUATION OF DENTAL PAIN

Of all the aspects of history taking, this is the one where a systematic approach is essential. The patient in pain can often be rambling and disjointed. The dentist must have a clear plan in mind and must bring the patient back to it by firm questioning.

The following questions are important:

- Where is the pain, i.e. tooth, gum, face, ear?
- Does it change position, i.e. radiate elsewhere?
- Describe the pain, e.g. throbbing, sharp, dull.
- How long has the pain been there?
- How strong is it?
- How long does it last?
- What brings it on?
- What takes it away?
- Does it come at any particular time — day or night?
- How often does it occur?
- Is it getting worse or getting better?
- Are there any associated symptoms, e.g. swelling, bad taste?

It can be useful to have the patient scale the intensity of the pain from one to ten and give some pictorial representation of the intensity, duration and frequency of each attack (Fig. 2.1).

Do not lead the patient; questions should be phrased so that a descriptive reply, rather than a plain 'yes' or 'no' is required. The description of the pain

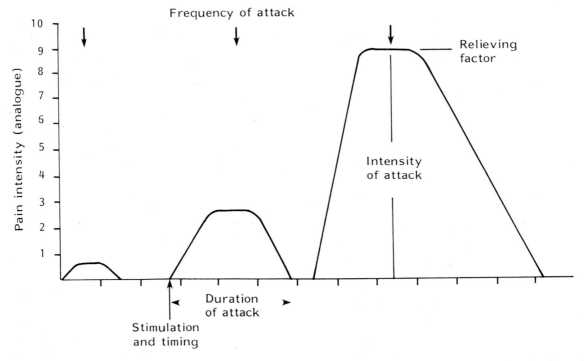

**Fig. 2.1** Schematic characterization of pain. The diagram shows the initiation of the pain, its frequency, intensity, duration and the effect of any relieving factors.

will lead to certain provisional diagnoses and also allow the exclusion of others.

## Pulpal disorders

The correlation of symptoms with actual pulp state is very poor. It is possible for several grades of pathology to be present within the same pulp. For instance, a single pulp could have an area of necrosis, an area of chronic pulpitis and an area of acute pulpitis (Ch. 6), but it would almost certainly be the acute pulpitis which provoked the painful symptoms. So bearing in mind the pitfalls of the precise diagnosis, the following generalizations about symptoms can be made.

### Physiological response

The pulp will respond to extremes of temperature through a sound crown, but the pain will be transient and stop as soon as the stimulus is removed.

When dentine is exposed by caries, trauma or simply gingival recession, then saliva and acid or alkali ions will reach the odontoblastic processes. The disturbance of the neutral pH will cause symptoms, usually of a transient and mild nature.

Temperature changes may stimulate pain, either when larger areas of cervical dentine are exposed, or when caries has spread well into the tooth. However, the pain stops when the stimulus is removed, though in *dentine hypersensitivity* the pain can be quite unpleasant.

Once toxins or bacteria reach the pulp, the symptoms become more severe.

### Acute pulpitis

The symptoms are classically an intense throbbing pain, initiated by heat, sometimes relieved by cold, well localized to one tooth, though sometimes radiating to the ear from the lower molar region. The patient is kept awake at night, and standard analgesics are not very effective. It is usually episodic, with increasing frequency and intensity of each episode, until it becomes continuous. It stops when the pulp dies or is removed.

*Chronic pulpitis/slow dying (moribund) pulp*

This condition often produces no symptoms, but may give rise to vague, dull and diffuse pain along a quadrant, i.e. it is poorly localized. Examination will often reveal several teeth with deep restorations, any one of which could be the cause.

### Apical infection

Chronic areas are usually symptomless, hence the need for continued radiographic review of root treated teeth. Acute apical periodontitis usually creates an intense throbbing pain, which is not affected by temperature, is fairly continuous, grows worse at night and is initiated or made worse by biting or knocking the tooth. It is usually well localized, and percussing the teeth for diagnostic purposes is unnecessary (and cruel). Routine analgesics are not very successful and the pain stops immediately once the pressure within the bone is relieved, usually when the infection has caused perforation of the cortical plate followed by formation of a soft tissue abscess, or sinus. If pressure builds up again in the soft tissues, then a throbbing pain is likely to recur but not as intense as that produced by the rigidly confined infection. In the latter case, *swelling* will be an accompanying complaint.

### Periodontal disease

General acute periodontal disease will give rise to generalized soreness of the mouth with perhaps bleeding gums, a bad taste and painful eating as accompanying symptoms.

Local conditions, such as pericoronitis or a lateral periodontal abscess, will cause more localized pain and soreness, particularly on eating.

Chronic periodontal disease is usually painless, but symptoms of bleeding or a bad taste are good indicators. Mild acute exacerbations sometimes occur as a result of occlusal trauma, and these cause vague diffuse pain, similar to the moribund pulp.

### Temporomandibular joint dysfunction and other facial pain

This is discussed in more detail in Chapter 20, but the clinician must be careful not to place the difficult diagnostic pain problem into this category for want of any better ideas. Remember that the **most common cause of pain** around the jaws arises from the pulp and the periodontal ligament and these must be investigated first.

Derangements and inflammation of the temporomandibular joint (TMJ) can lead to pain which is localized to the joint area, sometimes felt within the external auditory meatus, and usually accompanied by clicking or crepitus in the joint.

The more common symptoms arise from the muscles of mastication and give rise to facial pain and headaches. The pain is usually in the area of the affected muscles, though occasionally retro-orbital pain is described. The character of the pain is typical of all acute muscular problems — soreness, tenderness, difficulty with movement, and sometimes a clear starting point is remembered, such as a wide yawn, removal of wisdom teeth, etc.

Pain described outside the muscle areas may not be from TMJ dysfunction; for instance the maxillary antrum sometimes produces overlapping anterior pain. The most classic pain picture is that of *trigeminal neuralgia*, with its trigger zone and paroxysms of intense pain. However, this character can be modified into *atypical facial pain* which may be trigeminal in origin, psychotic or due to central nervous system lesions. Pain that crosses the midline is often psychotic in origin.

However, in all these cases, the purely dental causes must be eliminated first.

### Summary

A full description of the pain should be obtained which will undoubtedly lead to an incomplete provisional diagnosis. However, an open mind is important until after the clinical examination, so early categorization of pain should be avoided.

Caries tends to affect several teeth in the same mouth, and so these teeth could exhibit different stages of the pathology. Symptoms of each could co-exist in the same quadrant, and confuse the pain picture completely. Here each facet of the symptoms needs to be analysed separately.

## MEDICAL HISTORY

Information about the patient's general health is essential for the planning of his dental care. Some medical conditions will influence the component items of a treatment plan or change its whole direction, whilst others will influence the way in which care is delivered. This is discussed in detail in Chapter 4.

Past and present disease experience should be questioned together with information about current drug therapy. A structured series of questions is the most reliable way of taking a medical history (Table 2.1), but the questioner must be careful not to miss anything because the patient misunderstands or mishears the questions.

**Table 2.1**  Medical history taking

Have you ever suffered from:
  any serious disease?
  any heart or chest trouble?
  rheumatic fever, chorea or growing pains?
  pneumonia or bronchitis?
  jaundice or hepatitis?

Do you have:
  bleeding disorders?
  diabetes?
  epilepsy?

Have you ever had a blood transfusion?

Have you ever given blood, or been turned down as a donor?

Are you allergic to any drugs or antibiotics?

Have you ever taken penicillin, and were you alright after?

Have you ever been in hospital or had any operations?

Are you taking any tablets or medicines at the moment?

  (Watch out for anticoagulants, steroids, drug abusers etc)

Have you been ill or consulted your doctor recently?

## PREVIOUS EXPERIENCE OF DENTISTRY

The patient's previous experience will have conditioned him to expect certain things of dentistry in general. These could be good or bad. The patient's attitude, in turn, is conveyed to the dentist, who may respond by tailoring the treatment plan accordingly. The patient may have particularly high or low aspirations, depending upon his previous experience; the dentist will judge the extent of this previous experience and may be influenced to continue the same basic pattern.

The important aspects to question are:

- Range of treatment experience
- Method of delivery of care, e.g. sedation

- Experience of analgesia/anaesthesia
- Prostheses: age, comfort, function
- General satisfaction with previous care
- Any particular problems

The answers will indicate any special needs, such as non-adrenaline containing local analgesic, use of sedation and so on. The patient's opinion of his dentures will help the decision about possible replacement or relining.

A patient dissatisfied with his previous care could continue to be dissatisfied, even if the new dentist provides the best care possible. Unfortunately, dentistry and plastic surgery attract perfection seekers.

## FAMILY AND SOCIAL HISTORY

The general home and work environment may dictate how easy or difficult it might be to carry out oral hygiene procedures or maintain a non-cariogenic diet. The home might also contain entrenched attitudes to dental care.

Work patterns, e.g. shiftwork, absences from home, or the need to care for young children, may reduce the ability to attend for prolonged courses of treatment. Anxiety and emotional problems can be initiators of stress related facial pain and muscle disorders (Ch. 20).

## HISTORY TAKING — SUMMARY

The efficiency of history taking will be related to the confidence of the patient in the listening powers of the dentist and the ability of both to communicate with each other.

History taking should not be a rigid system of check lists, though there must be a consistent basis for the dentist's questions. The programme of questioning must be flexible and adapted towards the individual patient — it is his story.

## CLINICAL EXAMINATION

The clinical examination must establish the status of the oral tissues as a basis for diagnosis and treatment. It is important to observe and record health as well as disease, and to be as accurate as possible. These observations must be part of a continuing exercise which should be performed briefly at every visit, particularly over long courses of treatment, since nothing remains static.

Comprehensive, sequential, up-to-date and easily read records are necessary to assess the progress of conditions, particularly when a preventive approach is being used, e.g. application of fluoride to early enamel caries. A brief scan of the records should re-inform the dentist of the patient's background at each visit. Many minutes can be wasted in thumbing back over old entries, so updated summary sheets are essential. Reviewing the summary sheets will provide the background for each visit and the decisions to be made as problems occur.

The *extra-oral examination* will not only give clues about the patient's attitude to treatment, his motivation or underlying medical condition, but may also indicate clinical or technical difficulties such as loss of vertical dimension or mandibular deviations. These problems may be identified during history taking by the observant clinician.

Palpation of the mandibular borders, temporomandibular joints and possible sites of lymph node involvement may reveal early pathology.

*Intra-oral examination* should commence with the area of the main complaint, if the patient has one. Certainly if there is pain, then some form of stabilization will be necessary (Ch. 3), which could be prevented if time is taken for a full examination first.

The recording of caries and restorations is based on the use of the *dental chart*, which can easily become a static record. It is valuable as a record of the teeth and the planned restorations at the beginning of treatment but, as work proceeds, it becomes out of date. Periodic re-charting should be done so that there is not just a chart of the teeth some years ago, when the patient joined the practice, with line upon line of restored holes at each course of treatment, but a single current chart.

The examination of the teeth for caries and restoration defects should be done after a thorough *prophylaxis* to remove stains and debris which would otherwise obscure observation. A dry field and a good light are traditionally necessary, but a probe should only be used with caution. The probe should not be used to test a 'sticky fissure' since the application of pressure will simply break it down further. Occlusal caries should be diagnosed principally by appearance — darkness underlying the cuspal slopes — aided in the deeper lesions by

radiography (p. 11). Additionally, transillumination is useful for unrestored teeth, and this technique can also reveal cracks in the enamel.

The margins of existing restorations are difficult to examine, particularly approximally, without using a probe, because such areas cannot be seen clearly and may be obscured by the restoration on radiographs. The probe must, though, be used gently to avoid creating a defect which did not exist previously (Fig. 2.2).

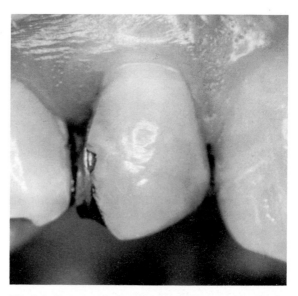

**Fig. 2.2** Recurrent caries around the disto-buccal margin of the amalgam restoration in 5⌋. This is shown by the fracture of the enamel margin and the white zone around the bucco-cervical corner.

Examination of the *periodontium* requires observation of gingival shape, size, texture and colour, and also crevice depth. Where the crevice is deeper than 3 mm, this would indicate pathology and a *pocket charting* is necessary. Exactly as the tooth chart, the periodontal chart must be redrawn periodically to record tissue response to therapy and oral hygiene measures. The chart must show gingival and bone levels from both buccal and lingual views.

In addition, diagnosis and treatment planning can be aided by the Community Periodontal Index of Treatment Needs (CPITN). The periodontium is probed with a World Health Organization CPITN probe to determine pocket depth, bleeding response

**Table 2.2** The CPITN analysis

| Clinical finding | Code | Treatment indicated |
|---|---|---|
| No disease | 0 | No treatment |
| Gingival bleeding after probing | 1 | Oral hygiene |
| Supra- or sub-gingival calculus | 2 | Scaling and oral hygiene instruction |
| Pockets 4–5 mm deep | 3 | Scaling and oral hygiene instruction |
| Pockets 6 mm and deeper | 4 | Scaling, oral hygiene instruction and more complex treatment |
| No teeth in sextant | – | |

to detect calculus. The probe is light with a ball tip of 0.5 mm diameter that is designed to detect sub-gingival calculus without penetrating the floor of the pocket. The mouth is divided into sextants and the worst clinical finding in each is recorded as the code for that sextant. The findings and clinical implications are shown in Table 2.2.

An oral hygiene index is also a useful way of monitoring the patient's cleaning efficiency, for use in both the surgery and the home. A simple scoring of the amount of plaque on selected tooth surfaces, following disclosing, is recorded in the notes. There are several oral hygiene or debris indices, but the simplest is that of Greene and Vermillion, which uses six teeth, an upper and lower molar on opposite sides, an upper and lower premolar on opposite sides and an upper and lower incisor on opposite sides. Both lingual and buccal surfaces are scored by:

0 = no plaque present
1 = plaque present on cervical third
2 = plaque present on both cervical third and middle third
3 = plaque present on whole surface.

The index is the total scored, divided by the number of surfaces examined.

The precise examination and charting of the teeth and periodontium should be accompanied by the examination of the *oral mucosa* and *oro-pharynx*.

Examination of the *occlusion* is discussed in detail in Chapter 12, but briefly, arch form, missing teeth and their effects, and restoration of the occlusion by dentures, crowns and bridges should be assessed.

Centric occlusion, centric relation and lateral and protrusive movements should be observed and noted and, where appropriate, a diagnostic articulated mounting should be used.

## SPECIAL INVESTIGATIONS

### Pulp vitality testing

An indication of the condition of the pulp is of great diagnostic value, but the methods available fall far short of the absolute. Most methods rely on nerve stimulation by electricity, thermal change or mechanical interference, but really the vitality of a pulp depends on its blood supply, which cannot be tested easily.

Complications also arise because of the varying state of the tissues in a single diseased pulp. Multi-rooted teeth can have one root containing vital pulp, and the other containing necrotic debris, thus a false positive could be recorded. Pus or inflammatory exudate in the root canal can conduct electricity; this is another reason for a false positive result. False negative results can occur because the pulp is insulated by much secondary dentine, or because the enamel is unable to transmit the stimulus because of its thickness or its proximity to large restorations. Teeth restored with insulating materials, such as ceramics or polymers, are also difficult to test.

*Electric pulp testing* passes a low current at high potential through the tooth. The current must have a square wave form because it must pass through enamel and dentine, which are relatively poor conductors, and reach the other side at sufficient potential to stimulate the nerves of the pulp.

Unfortunately, numbers are ascribed to the patient's response, and this gives the test more apparent scientific validity than it actually possesses. In reality it is subjective, with a 'yes' or a 'no' as the response. The patient's expectation of the test influences the result, particularly if the sensation from the first, control tooth is very painful. A pre-emptive response is very likely in the subsequent tests.

Because false positive and false negative results are possible with electric pulp testing it should be complemented with *thermal tests* to increase the information available. Ice sticks or ice crystals, made by evaporating ethyl chloride, can be used but the amount of ice applied must be substantial to create sufficient temperature differential to affect the pulp. Because the tooth crown is a good heat sink, a small pledget of cotton wool with ice crystals may have no effect. Hot gutta percha or impression compound should be applied to a lubricated tooth surface to contrast with the cold results. Interestingly, the effect of heat is often less than that of cold since the temperature difference is larger when dropping from 37° to 0°C, compared with the rise from 37° to about 65°C.

The most reliable pulp test is the *test cavity*; this can be done quite simply by starting a cavity in the tooth under test, without local analgesia, and stopping as soon as there is a response. Non-operative pulp tests must be interpreted with caution, but they produce one more piece of the diagnostic jigsaw to be placed alongside the clinical examination and the radiographic findings.

## Blood tests

The oral tissues may be the first to reflect systemic disease and a full cell count and haemoglobin estimation may be indicated in cases of abnormal gingival inflammation to exclude blood dyscrasias such as leukaemia or anaemia. Examination for viral hepatitis B antibodies is essential with anyone giving a history of jaundice or hepatitis because of the special risks they present to the dentist and technical staff in relation to cross-infection (Ch. 4).

Patients on anticoagulant therapy may require a corrected prothrombin time (BCR) estimation prior to some forms of dental treatment and changes to therapy should only be made in consultation with the physician responsible. This, of course, requires support from the local hospital, and if this is not forthcoming, the treatment plan would have to be modified accordingly.

## RADIOGRAPHY

Radiographs are essential for proper diagnosis and treatment planning in conservative dentistry. Three views are important: the orthopantomogram (OPT/OPG), the bitewing and the periapical. The information they provide is as follows:

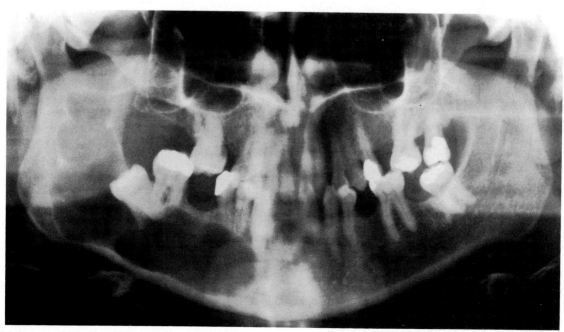

**Fig. 2.3** An orthopantomogram showing a large cystic lesion of the right ramus. The patient had been referred because of anterior attrition.

- OPT
    general scan of the teeth and jaws
    buried teeth, roots and cysts
    apical infection
    existence of root fillings
    TMJ (sometimes)
- Bitewing
    caries: approximal and occlusal
    depth of restorations
    restoration integrity
    interdental bone height
    pulp chamber morphology
- Periapical
    apical infection
    integrity of root fillings and posts
    interdental bone
    root fractures and perforations
    resorption
    root canal morphology

The value of the OPT as a routine scan for every new patient cannot be overstated. Figure 2.3 shows an OPT of a patient referred for attrition of the lower incisors!

However, the OPT does not give sufficient definition for the diagnosis of caries or for the accurate estimation of interdental bone height. In some areas, there may be masking of the root apices by overlapping structures, and occasionally apparent apical radiolucencies may be seen, which are in fact artefacts. In addition, because of variable image densities and the angulation of the beam in certain areas, dramatic mis-diagnoses are possible. Figure

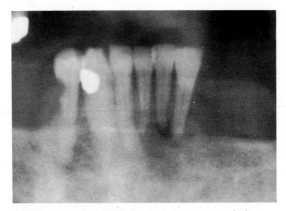

**Fig. 2.4** Part of an OPT showing an apparent apical radiolucency on 1|. Root canal therapy was started on the basis of this film.

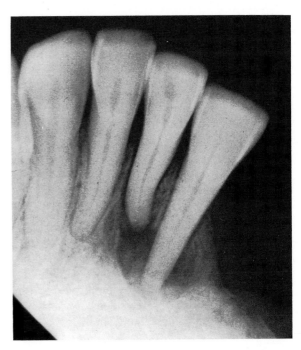

**Fig. 2.5** Apical film of the suspicious area in Figure 2.4. The radiolucency is centred on the |2, not arising from the apex and was found to be a lateral periodontal cyst.

2.4 shows part of an OPT which shows a very precise radiolucency, apparently associated with the lower left central incisor. Based on this film only, and without a vitality test, root canal therapy was started. The tooth was painful. An apical film was then ordered (Fig. 2.5) which suggested that the radiolucency was associated more with the lateral incisor than the central. The lateral incisor was vital to pulp testing. The radiolucency is not 'right' for an apical area — it is round, not merging smoothly with periodontal space and is higher than it should be. A surgical exploration was undertaken and the radiolucency turned out to be a lateral periodontal cyst.

Clearly then, bitewing and periapical films are required to confirm OPT findings and to show precise detail. The bitewing is more reproducible than the periapical because variations in tube angulation when taking periapicals are almost inevitable, even when the long cone technique is used. This leads particularly to differences in the definition of interdental bone.

It must be remembered that the radiograph is a two dimensional picture of a three dimensional

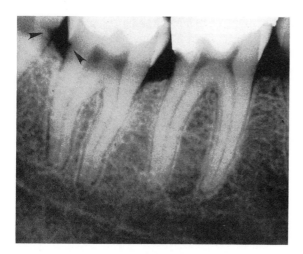

**Fig. 2.6** A periapical radiograph of $\overline{76|}$ showing cervical radiolucencies (arrowed) mesially on $\overline{8|}$ and distally on $\overline{7|}$ which are artefacts caused by the curvature of the teeth. Contrast these with the more clearly defined recurrent caries under the distal margin of $\overline{6|}$.

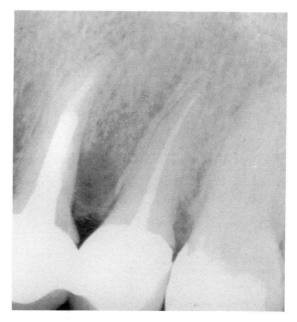

**Fig. 2.7** Periapical film of the $|\underline{5}$ showing a bridge retainer with apparently good adaptation at the distal margin.

entity and is dependent on mineral densities for its image. The depth of a carious lesion can be underestimated by as much as a third on a bitewing, and pulp horns can be superimposed on the caries, whereas they are actually in a different plane.

Root concavities, particularly in the approximal cervical areas may be shown as apparent areas of demineralization (Fig. 2.6).

Angulation is critical for both films when assessing restoration integrity. Unless the X-ray beam is precisely aligned along a cervical margin, the restoration will obscure the margin and appear sound (Figs. 2.7 and 2.8).

All radiographic findings should be confirmed wherever possible by repeating the clinical examination with the films alongside. Thus cervical overhangs or apparent approximal caries should be investigated by gentle probing. Summary sheets for radiographs taken and their findings should be an integral part of the notes, allowing easy reference and review. Of course, the quality of radiographs — both in the taking and the processing — has to be of the highest order for accurate conclusions to be made.

## SUMMARY

The meticulous collection and collation of all the information provided by the history, clinical

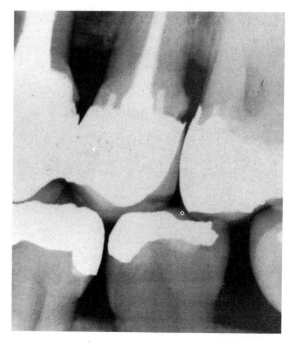

**Fig. 2.8** Bitewing film with its different angulation, reveals a deficiency of the distal margin.

examination, special tests and radiographs should provide the basis for the diagnosis and the treatment plan, and the continuing care of the patient. There can never be enough information, but care should be taken about guessing or taking things for granted. With clinical experience this might be acceptable, but for precision, the information must be accumulated as carefully and as fully as possible.

# 3. Diagnosis and stabilization

*P. H. Jacobsen*

The diagnosis is the summation and conclusions drawn from the assembly of all the separate pieces of information gathered from the patient's story, clinical observations, special tests and radiography (Fig. 3.1). It is an intellectual jigsaw puzzle which is completed as a list of pathological conditions and simple restorative disorders.

The *aetiology* of each condition should also be established so that this can be eliminated, if appropriate, to prevent recurrence of the problem.

In some cases, it will be necessary to carry out some operative investigation, either to confirm a *provisional diagnosis*, or to determine the actual diagnosis. For example, a deep carious lesion will usually need to be opened and investigated to reveal its extent, and to detect the presence of a pulpal exposure. Planning the restoration of such a tooth before investigation would be premature.

*Stabilization* is a series of procedures which is designed to control actively progressing pathology rapidly, to achieve:

- Pain relief
- Arrest of tissue destruction
- Final diagnosis
- The basis to plan the definitive management

The operative phase is instituted immediately, sometimes before the history and examination has been completed, so that no time is wasted in relieving symptoms. The treatment should be planned to be completed as quickly as possible and the procedures will be short and sharp, e.g. pulp extirpation, extraction.

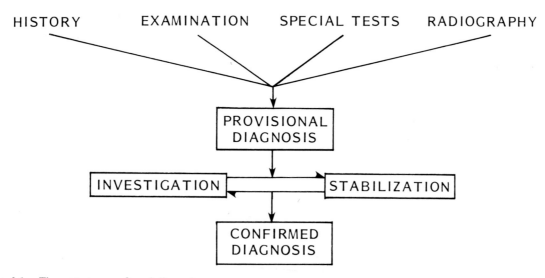

Fig. 3.1    The route to a confirmed diagnosis.

## DIAGNOSIS

### Caries

Some conditions are obvious; cavitation of the enamel coupled with a brown base and whitened edges usually indicates caries. Indeed, the jump from what is seen, to the diagnosis, is so rapid that the intermediate listing of physical signs is somewhat superfluous.

However, the aetiological factors may not be obvious. Is this one of many sites of *primary caries*, or an isolated *recurrent carious lesion* around a failing restoration? Is this the middle aged onset of *cervical caries* with its problems of rapid spread, or just fissure caries, which in some population groups would hardly qualify for a raised eyebrow?

So the *caries rate* is important, and the *Decayed, Missing and Filled (DMF)* score helps reflect this. But also the number of *active lesions* must be considered as an indication of the severity of the current pathology. *Diet analysis* would be appropriate for many patients with a high active caries rate, in order to determine the aetiology.

If it is an isolated recurrent lesion, this could be the result of operator error, and, if so, this must not be repeated on replacement of the restoration. Was it due to incorrectly sited margins, poorly finished enamel or the abuse of a matrix band (Fig. 3.2)? How deep has the caries spread around the restoration? Does the radiograph help, or is the lesion masked by the radiopacity of the amalgam? Only removal of the restoration and the caries will answer this.

### Restorations

The faults that can be diagnosed with long standing restorations are numerous. There could be corrosion, ditching and fracture of amalgam, or discolouration, marginal staining and surface loss of composite resin. There could be the technical faults of cervical overhangs, negative edges, incorrect occlusion, poor shade matching and perforations.

Having identified the fault, however, there is one very important question to be answered: has the fault induced any pathology? The reason for the question is that some faults are just minor technical errors or normal material behaviour, and to replace restorations purely for these reasons would be wrong.

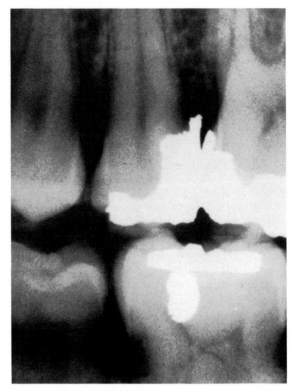

**Fig. 3.2** Bitewing radiograph showing recurrent caries at the disto-cervical aspect of |5, together with an overhanging amalgam margin.

Where pathology is associated with the fault, then clearly something must be done. Figure 3.3A shows ditched and corroded amalgams, which are technically less than pleasing, but in the absence of a positive diagnosis of associated pathology, they should not be replaced. Contrast them with that in Figure 3.3B and C, with its suspicious fracture line and underlying caries.

### Pulpal disorders

The history, pulp tests and radiography (Ch. 2) would have given some information about the possible state of the pulp. A deep carious lesion with no response to heat and cold, and electric pulp testing, together with apical radiolucency on radiograph, would lead to a certain diagnosis of *pulp necrosis* and *apical periodontitis*.

However, what about the painless deep lesion with an ambivalent pulp testing response and normal

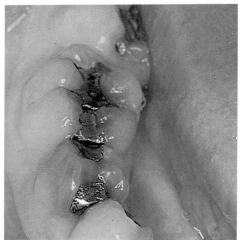

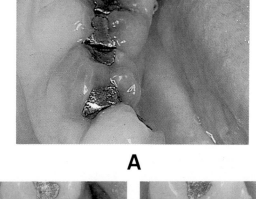

Fig. 3.3 **A**, Ditched and corroded amalgams, but still satisfactory restorations. **B**, Ditched and corroded occluso–palatal amalgam, but with a central fracture in it. This is much more suspicious. **C**, Removal of the amalgam revealed deep caries in two sites occlusally, together with a mesial lesion. The bitewing of this tooth (6|) (Fig. 9.12) was not very helpful.

apical anatomy on radiograph? Here it would be appropriate to make a provisional diagnosis of *chronic pulpitis* to be confirmed or refuted by operative investigation.

Episodes of intense pain, localized to one tooth, with the pain lasting after the initiating stimulus has been removed, with normal apical radiographic appearance would suggest *acute pulpitis*.

## Apical conditions

The diagnosis usually relies on the radiographic appearance of a radiolucent area at the root apex. For differential diagnostic purposes, a negative response to pulp testing is necessary to eliminate neoplasia,

such as cementoma, overlying fissural cysts, or simply an anatomical structure, such as a foramen.

If there are symptoms, and pain on percussion, then *acute apical periodontitis* is the diagnosis. A 'silent' apical area with a negative pulp test will be *chronic apical periodontitis*, an *apical granuloma* or an *apical cyst*. The differential diagnosis between these relies essentially on biopsy, as clinical and radiographic features do not distinguish them from each other.

Where the tooth is root filled and symptomless, an apical area may not be pathological, and serial radiographs are necessary to differentiate between a healing lesion and progressing pathology (Figs 3.4

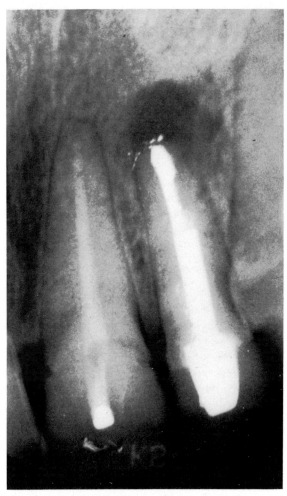

Fig. 3.4 Periapical radiograph of |2 immediately after apicectomy and retrograde root filling.

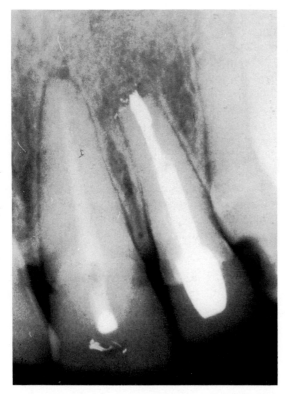

**Fig. 3.5** Complete apical in-fill of Figure 3.4. This took two years and the decreasing area shown on films taken in the meantime must be distinguished from apical pathology.

and 3.5). A static area may indicate healing by fibrous tissue without calcification, which would not be infected.

## Periodontal disease

The complaint of bleeding gums, the signs of reddened gingival margins with slight enlargement, and bleeding on probing with no pocket formation leads to the conclusion of the almost ubiquitous *chronic marginal gingivitis*.

But the severity of this, together with the amount of *plaque* and *debris* present, must accompany the diagnosis. Is there *hyperplasia* present as well, or just enlargement due to inflammatory oedema? Is the aetiology just *poor oral hygiene*, or are there other local factors such as faulty restoration margins which prevent the patient cleaning efficiently? Could there be *systemic* disorders, such as blood dyscrasias, present which modify the tissue response to the plaque?

Where soreness and even pain accompany the redness and bleeding, then an *acute gingivitis* may be present.

A *plaque index* is essential to accompany the diagnosis. Simple disclosing and the scoring of the extent of plaque coverage as described in Chapter 2 provides a good baseline against which to judge improvements.

The presence of a pathologically deepened gingival crevice, a *pocket*, and no pain indicates *chronic marginal periodontitis*. Radiographs, particularly bitewings, may reveal *vertical* or *horizontal bone loss* caused by the inflammation. Vertical bone loss leads to the diagnosis of an *infra-bony* pocket (Fig. 3.6).

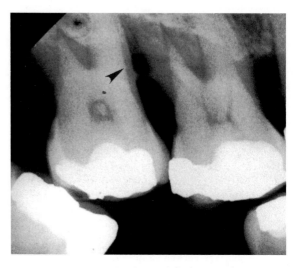

**Fig. 3.6** Radiograph showing an infra-bony pocket (arrowed) at 7|.

## Occlusal disorders

Impacted and malpositioned teeth are obvious diagnoses here. But also, the signs of occlusal derangement following tooth loss should be diagnosed. These are tilting, drifting and over-eruption of the adjacent teeth into the space, which, in turn, may bring pathology such as caries of approximal root surfaces, and periodontal disease from food impaction and plaque accumulation.

The inefficient restoration of the occlusion by dentures or crowns and bridges should be diagnosed, and the effects of occlusal interferences noted (Ch. 7).

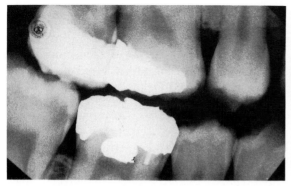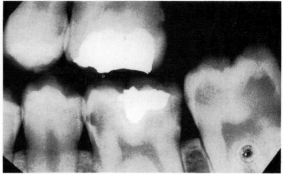

**Fig. 3.7**  Bitewing radiographs showing extensive caries which requires stabilization before definitive treatment is provided. There is deep primary caries in $\overline{7|67}$, recurrent caries cervically in $\overline{6|}$, and early lesions in almost all the other teeth.

## INVESTIGATION OF PROVISIONAL DIAGNOSES

The need for investigation in relation to the diagnosis of pulpal disorders has already been mentioned, but perhaps the most dramatic area where considerable investigation is necessary, is in the diagnosis of facial pain. Detailed description of the various conditions is outside the scope of this book, but there is a considerable overlap of the symptoms of caries and pulpitis, and those of sinusitis, TMJ dysfunction, trigeminal neuralgia and atypical facial pain. It is important to remember that the most common cause of pain around the lower face and jaws is pathology of the teeth and periodontium.

The dying or *moribund* pulp can produce the quite atypical symptoms of diffuse pain, unrelated to any stimulus, and radiating to areas served by the trigeminal nerve of the same side. The pulp will often be covered by a large, radio-opaque restoration, quite impervious to X-rays, and impossible to examine by non-invasive vitality tests. Worse still, because of the nature of caries, several of these restorations may exist together. It is essential that all these restorations are investigated thoroughly, before a committed diagnosis is made. It is very embarrassing to relieve long standing facial pain by the extraction of a non-vital tooth, when the patient has been taking tegretol for several months!

After careful clinical examination, pulp tests and radiographs, the next step is to remove individual restorations. This can be started without local analgesia as a very reliable mechanical pulp test. Explain the purpose of this to the patient, and that an analgesic will be given as soon as any pain is felt. Inspect the pulpal aspects of the cavity carefully, and if no exposure is found and the tooth is vital, place a sedative dressing.

Clinical experience will tend to suggest which teeth look suspicious, and which could be innocent.

## STABILIZATION

### Caries

Figure 3.7 illustrates a case of so-called *acute caries*. There is caries in most teeth, with some extensive loss of dentine. It would be quite wrong to approach the definitive restoration of $\overline{6|}$ first, find a carious exposure, root fill it, and then construct a pinned core and a full veneer crown. Whilst this was being done, the caries in the other teeth would be spreading ever onwards. So stabilization of the caries in the whole mouth is required.

The actual plan must be based on an overall assessment of the patient's expectations and the restorative possibilities. The extent of the caries does not reflect keen dental awareness. However, education is possible, if interest is there.

First, make an estimate of how many teeth could be restored simply, how many would require root canal therapy and how many would require crowns. Present this estimate and the implications of time and effort to the patient, and await the reaction. A keen, motivated reaction would suggest opening, investigating and dressing all the lesions, stabilizing the pulp as appropriate (p. 20), and extracting only those that are absolutely unrestorable. A disinterested reaction, on the other hand, would lead to extraction of those teeth whose prognosis was not assured after simple restoration, i.e. those with deep lesions.

## Acute pulpal and apical conditions

The most rapid and effective way of treating these, is to extract the tooth. The pulp is removed, and drainage of an apical abscess is very clearly established by this procedure.

However, if conservation of the tooth is indicated and root canal therapy is possible and it is restorable after such therapy, then rather different means must be used.

### Acute pulpitis

This should be stabilized by pulp extirpation. However, this may not be straightforward, since local analgesia may be sometimes difficult to achieve. This difficulty may be related to the persistence of the pain stimulus altering the nerve impulse conduction and making blocking by analgesic more difficult.

The first alternative is to repeat the local analgesic injection, but use a different agent. For instance, if xylocaine was given first, repeat with prilocaine. The two agents potentiate each other. Do not use more than three cartridges of xylocaine in any event. If this does not work, apply a topical corticosteroid paste to the exposed dentine. This will reduce inflammation and ease pain, and in 48 hours or so the patient should return for another attempt under local analgesic. Failing all these, the pulp will have to be extirpated under a general anaesthetic.

Ideally, the pulp should be extirpated from the full length of the root canal, so that remnants are not left behind which continue the pain. However, a diagnostic radiograph is necessary to assure this, and the duration of analgesia may not be long enough to allow it. If only partial extirpation has been achieved, apply a topical corticosteroid as a root canal dressing and complete the extirpation at the preparation stage. Total extirpation should be followed by root canal dressing with calcium hydroxide in propylene glycol.

### Apical periodontitis and apical abscess

This diagnosis presumes pulp necrosis and the presence of infection or leakage of toxins beyond the root apex. The canal must be cleared of debris and drainage established for the apical exudate, whose build-up causes the pain.

If an abscess has formed, then cutting an endodontic access cavity will be rewarded by pus leaking from the tooth. Pain relief can be instantaneous. If no pus or exudate appears, then a barbed broach should be used, well short of the apex, to clear any obstruction. If drainage is still not achieved, then passage of a fine (No. 8) file through the apical foramen must be considered. This diameter will establish drainage, but will not create the later difficulties in root filling caused by larger apical perforations.

The use of local analgesic should be cautious in the presence of acute inflammation. Restriction of the blood supply to the area could result in spread of the infection. Also the local analgesic may not be effective.

It is best to use an air turbine as much as possible to reduce vibration, and support the tooth, perhaps with a composition splint at the same time. Use a conventional speed handpiece to break the final half-millimetre or so.

If an abscess has pointed in the sulcus, this should be incised. Hot salt water mouthwashes should be used to apply heat to the alveolus and drainage should be maintained by the patient sucking the tooth to keep the access clear.

**Systemic antibiotics.** These should be restricted to cases where systemic involvement is apparent (i.e. raised temperature, malaise, tender regional lymph nodes) or where there is some medical indication. In these circumstances, two high doses of oral amoxycillin are very effective: 3 g immediately and 2 g 24 hours later.

**Review.** Drainage should be restricted to 24–48 hours. After this, more will go up the canal, than will come down. To complete the stabilization, the canal must be fully prepared (Ch.11). The reason for this is that the walls of the root canal will be infected (in contra-distinction to the acute pulpitis case) and simply irrigating and sealing the canal will not remove the infection.

## Traumatic injuries to the teeth

The immediate objective is the relief of pain and the procedure required will depend upon the site of any fracture and the state of the pulp. The pulp, however, can be concussed by a blow and may not provide a pulp test response for some weeks. Therefore, immediate stabilization must be followed by review for definitive diagnosis and management.

A complete history is essential in case of future litigation regarding the cause of the accident. All teeth in the area of the trauma should be pulp tested and radiographed, and if there are any soft tissue lacerations and missing tooth fragments, the tissues should be radiographed also. Where there is any doubt on the whereabouts of fragments, the possibility of facial fractures, or any general injury the patient should be referred to the local casualty department for complete investigation.

The treatment schemes for traumatized teeth are summarized below and for more detailed consideration the reader is referred to a specialized text.

### Enamel only fracture

Small fracture areas can simply be smoothed, whilst larger defects, which may affect aesthetics or function, should be restored with acid etch retained composite resin. The teeth should be reviewed in four to six weeks and the pulp tests and radiographs repeated. Negative pulp tests then may indicate that root canal therapy is necessary.

### Enamel/dentine fracture

**Superficial.** The tooth should be dressed with zinc oxide/eugenol cement in a temporary crown to aid pulp recovery. The crown must allow access to enamel for later pulp testing. If vital at review, then an acid etch retained composite resin restoration should be placed. Non-vitality would probably indicate root canal therapy.

**Deep.** These should be treated as pulp exposures.

### Enamel/dentine/pulp fractures and deep enamel/dentine fractures

With these the pulp is unlikely to recover and the management depends on whether the root apex has closed or is still open.

**Root formation complete.** Conventional root canal therapy is indicated plus semi-permanent restoration of the crown, usually by composite resin. A post crown should be avoided if at all possible, especially for young patients playing contact sports.

**Root apex open.** Root formation should be encouraged to finish. If the pulp is vital, *pulpotomy* is used to remove the coronal pulp, leaving radicular pulp to continue root formation. If the pulp is non-vital, the canal should be carefully filed short of the apex, and filled with calcium hydroxide in propylene glycol. This material creates conditions favourable for root formation. In both cases, when the apex has closed, the canal should be root filled.

If the apex does not close, then root canal therapy should be done — this is technically difficult (Ch. 11).

### Root fractures

**Apical third.** If symptomless and vital, these should be left and reviewed. Otherwise, they should be root filled to the fracture line and reviewed. If there is evidence of pathology the apical fragment should be removed.

**Middle third.** If the coronal fragment is mobile, it should be splinted to the adjacent teeth. In the absence of symptoms or pathology, it may be possible to place a post through both fragments to increase stability. If the fragments are not in line, this will not be possible, and the tooth should be root filled to the fracture line, and reviewed. The fragment may need to be removed and it is possible to use a long post extending into the bone as an implant to increase the stability of the crown. The prognosis for the middle third root fracture is poor.

**Coronal third.** The prognosis depends on the extent to which the fracture goes beyond the epithelial attachment, usually palatally. A very oblique fracture will be difficult to restore, and the tooth should be extracted.

A more shallow fracture would indicate root filling and the provision of a cast post and diaphragm to prevent root splitting later. The immediate stabilization is to extirpate the pulp and provide a temporary crown. The easiest way to do the crown is to use the tooth fragment and to acid etch it to the adjacent teeth, over the sealed root access.

*Dislocation and avulsion*

The dislocated tooth can be repositioned and splinted for about a week. Pulp recovery is unlikely and the root canal treatment should be done whilst the splint is in place.

The avulsed tooth can be replanted, but the success of this depends on the length of time it has been out of the mouth and how it was stored during that time. Milk is probably the best storage medium, though a parent could keep the tooth in their own buccal sulcus to be kept moist by saliva.

Before replanting, the tooth should be washed in normal saline, but no other cleaning should be done. The tooth should be splinted in place and root canal therapy carried out whilst the splint is on. It is unwise to leave the root canal empty. Calcium hydroxide has been shown to inhibit resorption, and this can be left in the canal for some time, with periodic replacement. The splint should be removed after a week.

*Review*

A traumatized tooth will require regular review by radiography, and if vital, pulp tests. Slow dentine formation can be induced by trauma, leading to the obliteration of the canal and difficult root canal therapy. If this is seen, the tooth should be root filled immediately whilst it is still possible. Late loss of vitality is also possible.

The other main complication of trauma is root resorption, either internal or external. This can sometimes be arrested by calcium hydroxide being placed in the canal. The periodontal ligament is replaced by ankylosis of the tooth to bone, and the tooth can remain firm for many years even though it has little root (Fig. 3.8). If infection supervenes, the tooth will require extraction.

## Acute gingival conditions and severe chronic periodontal disease

Acute gingival conditions should be treated by mouthwash and systemic antibiotics appropriate to the causative organism. In the presence of severe

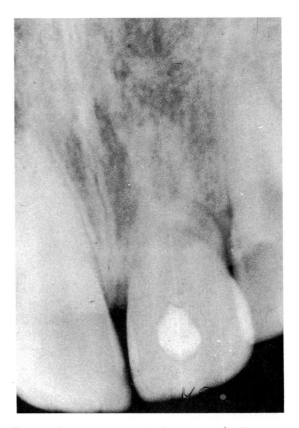

**Fig. 3.8**  Periapical radiograph of a replanted |1. The tooth has undergone external resorption, but is still firm due to ankylosis.

chronic periodontal disease, the gingivae must be stabilized before commencing restorations. Indeed a complete diagnosis of the state of the crowns could be impossible before resolution of gingival tissues (Fig. 3.9).

If the supporting tissues are not healthy, most restorative work will be impossible because of gingival bleeding or exudate, or incorrect level of the gingival margin. Scaling and polishing, and instruction in oral hygiene is required first, followed by review.

However, if the standard of the existing restorations is contributing to plaque retention, then the faulty ones should be removed, and well fitting provisionals placed, pending resolution of the gingival problems.

Intracoronal cavities can be provisionally restored with polycarboxylate cement, placed with the aid of a matrix, or even amalgam. This will provide the better

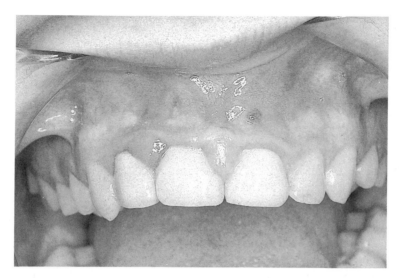

**Fig. 3.9**   Chronic marginal hyperplastic gingivitis associated with crowns on 21|1. The crowns must be corrected before the gingivae will resolve.

gingival and contact area contour. Replacement of the temporary amalgams should be done after resolution of the soft tissue inflammation.

## SUMMARY

1. Draw conclusions from the history and examination — the diagnosis;

2. If the data are inconclusive, make a provisional diagnosis;
3. Investigate to confirm the diagnosis;
4. Control active pathology as rapidly as possible;
5. When stable, draft the definitive treatment plan.

# 4. Treatment planning

*P. H. Jacobsen*

The treatment plan is the basic blueprint for the delivery of care. It combines priorities for therapy with the organization and management of that therapy. It must combine *prevention* of disease with the eradication and repair of pathology.

The treatment plan must fit the profiles of both the patient and the dentist (Fig. 4.1). As was discussed in Chapter 1, the patient will have some ideas about his dental future, and the dentist will have certain resources and technical skills available to fulfill treatment objectives. Basically, the resources available, governed by the dentist's tech-

niques should, through the medium of the treatment plan, match the resource consumption of the patient, governed by his expectations and his pathology.

Figure 4.2 projects the patient from diagnosis, through agreement and formal *consent* to the treatment and its delivery, to oral health and the very important concept of *continuing care*.

To a large extent, the left side of Figure 4.1 will be dealt with in the succeeding chapters, and problems created by the patient himself will be considered here.

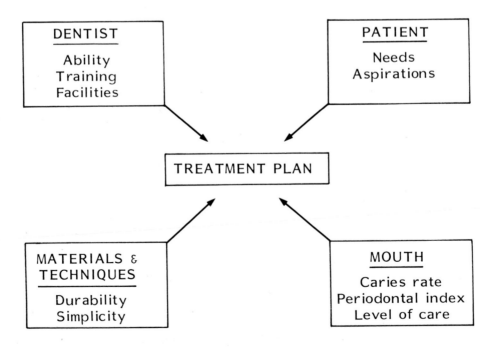

**Fig 4.1** The factors influencing a treatment plan.

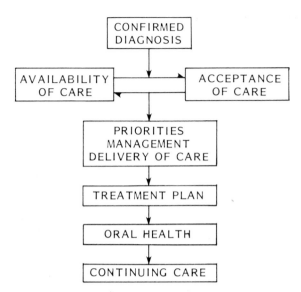

**Fig 4.2**  The route to oral health and continuing care.

## THE PATIENT'S INFLUENCE ON TREATMENT PLANNING

### Motivation, expectations and availability

These go hand in hand — a well motivated patient will almost always find a way to make himself available for treatment. A string of failed appointments belies initial protestations of interest and desire for treatment.

If there are doubts about the patient's commitment, then this should be reflected in a cautious start to the treatment plan. One or two visits to the hygienist, followed by a short appointment with the dentist for a simple restoration and review of oral hygiene would be appropriate. Provided active pathology has been stabilized, then the weaker patient might well benefit from a repeated oral hygiene lesson, together with the message that unless oral hygiene improves, restorative work will not be started. Certainly, this must be the case prior to advanced restorations.

As was discussed earlier, the extraction of a tooth may fit a patient's expectations more than attendance for four or five visits for root canal therapy and a crown. It may be that the conservative treatment is well within the dentist's capabilities, but it will be wasted if the patient loses interest after the first hour, when the root canals are being identified. Of course, this is not to suggest that the dentist should not try

to educate and inform about restorative possibilities. It could be that the patient never realized the scope of modern dentistry. However, initial enthusiasm must be maintained so that it is not just the product of the dentist's ambitions.

### Apprehension

No one likes visiting the dentist, mainly in view of the prospect of minor surgery to a very tender area of the anatomy, but also because of the folklore surrounding the profession.

The majority of those who actually come for treatment are able to control their apprehension successfully, but a minority have tremendous difficulty. Often, their apprehension stems from a single unpleasant experience, perhaps as a child, and frequently pain from poor analgesia is remembered vividly. Many of these will respond to sympathetic listening, careful explanations about treatment, an unhurried, relaxed chairside manner and a great deal of patience.

Simple procedures with complete analgesia should be done first to establish confidence, and then more complex work may be possible. The more intractable cases may be candidates for inhalation sedation, intravenous sedation or general anaesthesia.

#### Inhalation sedation

This technique involves the administration of 25% nitrous oxide at flow rates in excess of the patient's minute volume requirements. The patient, therefore, breathes a gas mixture of constant concentration and becomes able to predict its effects. He can then regulate the amount of sedation he takes as required.

The gas is administered through a nose piece and the patient can chose to breathe the gas through the nose, or take in air through the mouth. Unconsciousness is impossible at the 25% level, which cannot be exceeded. Slightly higher levels, even 28%, can lead to unconsciousness in some patients. The other advantages of the low concentration are that pharyngeal reflexes are not depressed and it is not necessary to starve patients prior to treatment.

The operator must encourage and reassure the patient during induction and treatment. There is certainly an element of hypnosis in the procedure.

Local anaesthesia must be used for painful procedures.

It is not possible to use inhalation sedation if the nasal airway is obstructed, the patient cannot lie supine or is in the first eight weeks of pregnancy.

Inhalation sedation should not be confused with *relative analgesia*, which uses somewhat higher concentrations of nitrous oxide and therefore is potentially more dangerous. Unconsciousness is possible and the patient would not be able to leave the surgery unaccompanied, or to drive.

## Intravenous sedation

A few patients are not able to respond to inhalation sedation, and for these the administration of a sedative intravenously is usually successful. Modern, short-acting benzodiazepines such as midazolam, are very suitable for outpatient sedation. Midazolam has a very short half-life and therefore a short recovery period. It also induces amnaesia, which can be very helpful.

The patient should not have eaten for 4–6 hours before the sedation is begun, but may drink small quantities after that. No alcohol should be taken, but regular medication should be taken as usual. Any anxiolytics will probably reduce the dose of sedation required. The drug is best administered through an in-dwelling venous cannula in the antecubital fossa, hand or forearm. The patient should be supine and the drug injected slowly at 2 mg (1 ml) every minute.

The patient should be observed continuously and sedation is adequate when:

- The patient looks relaxed
- He has slow or slurred speech
- Verrill's sign (eye half-covered by eyelid) is present

Communication is important as the patient will respond slowly to command. Local analgesia is also necessary. If the sedation becomes less, then a further increment titrated against response, should be given.

After the treatment is completed, recovery should be observed and the patient can go home escorted, when he is lucid and capable of walking unaided. The patient must avoid driving, sport and alcohol for 12 hours.

## General anaesthesia

Intubated general anaesthesia in day stay facilities should be reserved for those who cannot be treated in any other way. It may also be appropriate for stabilizing urgent cases who will subsequently have definitive treatment under inhalation sedation.

It is really the last resort and is a compromise because of the limited time available — say, about an hour — and the difficult working conditions of an operating theatre. Only very basic conservation should be planned and any teeth of dubious prognosis should be extracted.

The patient should be screened by haemoglobin estimation, blood count, urinalysis and blood pressure to ensure fitness for anaesthesia. They must be starved and not have any acute respiratory infections. Patients with medical problems should be admitted for observation before and after the anaesthetic.

Care must be taken during treatment not to flood the pharynx with water and to ensure all pieces of tooth, amalgam, etc. are removed from the mouth.

The patient must be accompanied home and looked after for 24 hours. They should return for a normal outpatient appointment for review and occlusal adjustment of restorations, which is not possible in theatre.

Many patients dislike the experience so much that they are very susceptible to conversion to less traumatic techniques.

## The influence of medical history on treatment planning and management

The taking of the medical history and its importance was outlined in Chapter 2. Medical conditions may influence the content of the treatment plan and/or the way in which care is delivered. For example, some conditions may indicate the extraction of a tooth rather than its restoration, whilst others may indicate that restorations, planned normally, are carried out under special conditions.

## Cardiovascular conditions

Probably the most confusion arises from the influence of a history of *rheumatic heart disease*.

Transient *bacteraemias* may lead to bacteria colonizing scarred areas of the endocardium, usually the valve edges, causing *bacterial endocarditis*. Bacteraemias occur every day from chewing or defecation, and certain dental procedures may cause them.

However, the relationship between dental procedures and the development of bacterial endocarditis is circumstantial only, since the confirmed diagnosis of the disease may take several months. The history of a previous dental procedure could just be coincidental. Couple this with the number of people who have had no antibiotic cover for many years of dentistry, including extractions, with no ill effects and the rationale for special management is less than convincing.

The nationally agreed recommendations are, though, to provide antibiotic cover for susceptible patients for dental procedures which carry a high risk of major bacteraemia. These procedures are:

- Extractions
- Scaling and polishing
- Surgery involving the gingival margin

There is no proof that endodontic procedures are incriminated in the aetiology of endocarditis, though care must be taken to remain within the confines of the root canal. (This is true for all root canal therapy, anyway.)

The definition of the susceptible patient is more difficult. Not all patients who give a history of rheumatic fever will have scarred endocardia, revealed by the presence of a murmur. To prescribe antibiotics for these patients would appear to be wasteful, if not a misuse of antibiotics. It is safer to request an opinion from a medical practitioner, preferably a cardiologist, as to whether cover is indicated.

Other cases where cover is definitely indicated are where there is a previous history of endocarditis, presence of a prosthetic heart valve or congenital cardiac defects.

The regime for prophylaxis is now based on a single high dose of amoxycillin (3 g preoperatively), or two high doses of erythromycin (1.5 g preoperatively and 0.5 g postoperatively). There are further recommendations for high risk patients (see Bibliography).

For dental procedures which do not carry a high risk and for which antibiotic cover should not be prescribed, such as gingival retraction or the placing of a matrix band, the gingival margin should be cleaned with an antiseptic, such as chlorhexidine.

All patients in the at-risk groups should be informed of the need to maintain good oral hygiene and those patients who are candidates for cardiac surgery should be well restored first.

*Treatment planning*

The healthy patient, with a history of rheumatic fever, should be treatment planned as normal. The higher risk patient, particularly if there is a history of endocarditis, should be planned more radically. A tooth requiring a possibly difficult root filling should be extracted, and any areas of chronic infection should be regarded with suspicion, and the teeth not given the benefit of the doubt.

Other cardiovascular conditions may make prolonged courses of treatment risky or difficult. This group includes stroke and cardiac infarction. Full recovery from such an episode, of course, should bring no problems, though the dentist ought to be prepared for a recurrence in the chair and for the management of collapse. For those patients with incomplete recovery, treatment should be planned to be simple, and provided in short appointments. The trauma from extraction should be avoided if at all possible. Stroke patients with residual paralysis may need advice on oral hygiene aids, such as electric toothbrushes.

## Blood borne viruses and the prevention of cross-infection

The two most important blood borne viruses in dentistry are hepatitis B virus (HBV) and human immunodeficiency virus (HIV).

Patients who are ill with hepatitis B or AIDS should receive dental treatment under hospital conditions. Those people who are known to be infectious, but are well, may be treated in normal dental practice and should be treatment planned as normal. Many carriers are unidentified, and these are treated unknowingly as normal patients. These and the known ones constitute a joint hazard to the dentist and other staff, and to the patients following them in the surgery.

The basic routine for the prevention of cross-infection should be applied to all patients, and the recommendations are referred to in the bibliography. In brief, the key recommendations are:

1. Protection of the operator and close-support dental surgery assistant by gloves, masks and glasses;
2. Effective decontamination and sterilization of all instruments and equipment which have touched the patient or have been handled by 'contaminated' staff;
3. Use of disposable equipment wherever possible;
4. Use of precise surgery routines to avoid contaminating areas, such as inside drawers or the stock of temporary crowns, which will be difficult to sterilize later;
5. Cleaning of contaminated surgery surfaces and their protection using tray systems and cling film;
6. Decontamination of all items to enter the laboratory.

When the patient is known to be a carrier, then the above recommendations must be followed together with more rigorous personal and surgery protection and cleaning. Again, the reader is referred to the bibliography for further information.

*Other medical conditions*

*General infirmity* or *terminal illness* would indicate a minimum of complex work being attempted. The plan should be to stabilize sources of pain and discomfort as simply as possible.

*Blood dyscrasias* and *diabetes* may give rise to gingival problems because of the reduced resistance to infection and these will preclude anything but stabilization being carried out. The medical condition should be resolved prior to definitive conservation.

The operator would wish to conserve teeth wherever possible in *epileptics* to avoid dentures, in *haemophiliacs* to avoid extractions, and in cases with *irradiated bone* where post extraction healing can be prolonged and difficult. It is important to see patients before radiotherapy, whenever possible, to remove any teeth of dubious prognosis.

Altered management of a normal treatment plan would be appropriate for a controlled diabetic, where treatment is best carried out immediately after a meal when the blood sugar is higher.

Conservation for *pregnant* patients requires some minor modifications. The generally held view is that invasive procedures are best avoided in the first and third trimesters, and radiography avoided totally in the first. However, where urgent treatment is required, this should be done in any event. It is also important to complete treatment and reach stability in the second trimester, so that treatment is not required later when the patient will be uncomfortable, or immediately after the baby is born, when the mother will have other priorities.

### Level of previous care

The well restored and cared-for mouth encourages more of the same. It indicates the patient's desire for continuing care and his ability to maintain restorations in plaque free and caries free conditions.

Unfortunately, the quality of the previous restorative care, rather than its volume, can also modify a treatment plan. If the restorative work has not been provided to a high standard then, even though the patient has been a regular attender, the sheer volume of replacement work required may inhibit a totally restorative approach (Fig. 4.3).

Several missing teeth and a partial denture might well lead to extraction of a difficult restorative problem and its addition to the denture.

### Oral hygiene and periodontal disease

A high active caries rate may dictate extractions and simple restorations only, and generalized periodontal disease might indicate the same. Oral hygiene must be effective before advanced restorations are contemplated.

### Occlusion

Evidence of deterioration in occlusal relationships following tooth loss would indicate bridges or partial dentures (Ch. 15). Inadequate occlusion on bridges or dentures might indicate their replacement.

Premature contacts or non-working interferences might suggest occlusal equilibration (Ch. 12).

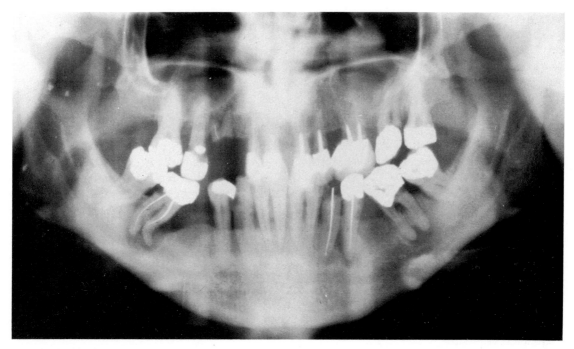

**Fig. 4.3** Orthopantomogram of a patient who has experienced extensive restorative dentistry. There is now gross caries and periodontal disease. The chances of success for future work are small, and, in any case, the volume of work required is daunting. The patient was treatment planned for a clearance and full dentures.

## Radiographic findings

The major use of radiography is in diagnosis (Ch. 2). However, it is absolutely essential in the planning of endodontics. The presence of patent root canals, absence of obstruction by secondary dentine, pulp stones or curvature can only be decided by good radiographs.

Having diagnosed acute pulpitis clinically, the radiograph will lead the planner to contemplate root canal therapy, or to recommend extraction. It might be very desirable to save the tooth, but it might be technically impossible.

## THE GENERAL STRUCTURE OF A TREATMENT PLAN

### Priorities

The simple treatment plan designed to treat chronic gingivitis, caries and failed restorations would begin by preparing the supporting tissues for restorative work (scaling and polishing, and preventing the recurrence of gingivitis) and instructing the patient in oral hygiene. This phase is better carried out by the dental hygienist, leaving the dentist free to perform more complex functions.

The priorities for simple restorations would relate to size, doing the largest first, unless the periodontium was being influenced by a poor contact area or over-hanging margin.

Oral hygiene should be reviewed continually during treatment with encouragement, or further reminders if necessary. If advanced work (crowns or endodontics) is planned, this should be placed at the end of the plan after gingival resolution and the completion of simple restorations. Oral hygiene review should also be satisfactory.

Extractions are best regarded within the framework of stabilization, since the affected teeth could give rise to pain whilst other work is being done. Also there is the possibility of damaging new restorations during surgery, particularly of impacted teeth. If the patient is to be referred for oral surgery, then this should be arranged early, but almost certainly the work will not be carried out until after the general practitioner has completed other treatment. At the time the referral is made, it is important to include information on proposed treatment of other teeth, so that the referring practitioner's responsibilities are established.

Any surgery involving the gingival margin, e.g. apicectomy, should be done well in advance of crowns or veneers proposed for the affected teeth.

Partial denture planning should be built in alongside the planning of restorations since the design may require rest seats, or specially modified crowns.

## Structure

A schematic arrangement for a treatment plan could be:

1. Prepare supporting tissues — scale and polish
2. Preventive measures — topical fluoride, fissure sealing, oral hygiene instruction, dietary advice
3. Design bridges or partial dentures
4. Simple restorations
5. Pinned restorations
6. Root canal therapy
7. Review oral hygiene and periodontal condition
8. Periodontal therapy, if necessary — root planing, surgery
9. Crowns
10. Construct dentures/bridges
11. Recall.

## REVIEW AND RECALL

The simple treatment plan has within its structure the review of oral hygiene procedures, but some other procedures would require formal review prior to progress in treatment. For example, apical surgery should not be followed immediately by crowns on the affected teeth. Two or three months should elapse whilst the gingival tissues stabilize and the margins reach a constant level, and an indication of apical healing is apparent.

Extractions and alveolar remodelling should be followed by review, perhaps six months later, before permanent bridges are considered.

The listing of a formal *recall* as part of the treatment plan is essential to indicate the responsibility for *continuing care*. The actual recall interval can be decided as appropriate to the patient's condition. Six months would be routine for most patients to monitor their plaque control and caries status, and to check for other oral pathology. Shorter intervals would be necessary for those having difficulties, whilst the well maintained patient could be left to their own devices for as long as a year.

Radiographic review of crowns and endodontics is essential. Symptomless loss of vitality under a crown preparation must be detected by the apical condition changing. Progressing healing of an apical lesion following root canal therapy should be monitored. The intervals can get progressively longer; beginning at six months, then a year later and two to three years regularly after that.

## SUMMARY

1. Decide on items for prevention and treatment;
2. Order these according to priority in the patient as a whole;
3. Review oral hygiene and prevention;
4. Break long treatment plans into stages, and review progress after each, to confirm that the next stage is appropriate;
5. Recall to commit the patient to continuing care.

# The restoration and its environment

# 5. Applied biology of the teeth

## D. K. Whittaker

Caries is a microbially initiated disease causing localized destruction of mineralized tissues in the body, including bone. For the purpose of this book only caries of the teeth will be considered and the signs of presence of the disease will be described as the localized destruction of enamel, dentine and more briefly, of cementum. As is the case with other pathological conditions, a clear understanding depends upon a knowledge of the basic structure of the tissues involved. In addition, restoration of tooth structure also depends on the same knowledge of the tissues against which the material is to be placed. The purpose of this chapter is to provide such information, to relate it to the environment surrounding the teeth and to discuss the implications for the restorative dentist.

## ENAMEL STRUCTURE AND CHEMISTRY

Enamel is the outer protective covering of the crown of the tooth and is an extremely hard, brittle, white, shiny substance. It is composed of billions of crystals of hydroxyapatite, which are roughly octagonal in cross-section, with a diameter of about 360 nm. The length of the crystals has proved difficult to determine but they are thought to be long and ribbon-like, extending for some distance through the enamel. The crystals are tightly packed together so that organic matrix lying between them is minimal, constituting only about 2% by weight of the enamel but much more than this by volume. Between the crystals are micropores or pores, the size of which can be measured with some accuracy, and changes in these spaces is one of the indications of the presence of carious attack. Under these conditions the enamel is said to have increased

porosity. The methods available for such studies will be discussed in Chapter 6.

### Prisms

The crystals of enamel are not randomly arranged but are grouped together to form rods or *prisms* of material, extending from the enamel-dentine junction to the surface of the tooth. In the original English literature the preferred term is that of 'prisms' whereas in more recent writings the term 'rod' is preferred and in fact induces a clearer image of the structure in the mind of the reader. Because the remainder of this book will use the word 'prism', the old-fashioned term will be used here.

Each prism has a mean cross-sectional diameter of about 5 $\mu$m but, because the surface area of the outer enamel is greater than that of the enamel dentine junction, the prisms tend to increase in diameter from the junction to the outer surface. The cross-sectional shape of the prisms has been variously described as octagonal, fish scale or keyhole shaped, but this depends to some extent on the angle of section. The keyhole concept is the classical construction in human enamel and is shown diagramatically in Figure 5.1. The broad part of the key hole is often referred to as the head and the narrow part as the tail. There is controversy as to what constitutes the boundary of each prism. Current research suggests that prism boundaries may be formed both by sudden changes in hydroxyapatite crystal orientation and by an increased concentration of *organic matrix*.

### Matrix

The nature of the organic matrix has received much

33

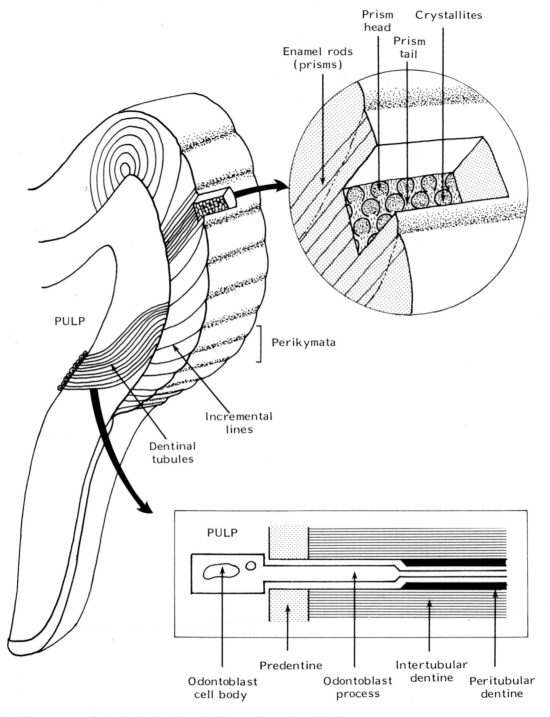

**Fig. 5.1**   The structure of a tooth, showing the main features of enamel and dentine.

attention, but because of its small amount has proved difficult to analyse with certainty. In the immature tooth the matrix consists of two distinct proteins — amelogenin and enamelin, and during maturation much of the amelogenin is removed. The cells responsible for secreting and maturing the enamel during development are the *ameloblasts* and they migrate outwards from the putative enamel–dentine junction for a distance equal to the thickness of the enamel at that point on the tooth.

When the ameloblasts have completed their secretory activity the final thickness of the enamel is determined and this cannot be increased throughout life, since the ameloblasts then degenerate. In principle enamel is a dead tissue which cannot repair itself. However, we will see later that chemically speaking some repair or re-structuring of enamel is possible.

### Incremental nature

The enamel is laid down by the ameloblasts in increments, arranged rather like the layers in an onion over each cusp of the tooth. In cross-section these appear as concentric rings through the enamel and are known as *incremental lines* or brown striae of Retzius (Fig. 5.1). Each line represents the point which the ameloblasts had reached at a particular time in their functional activity. The incremental line is not pigmented as the name would suggest but is probably caused by a slight change in direction and diameter of the enamel prisms. These incremental lines reach the surface of the tooth at an acute angle and there is evidence that they modify the progression of caries in the natural lesion.

### Surface structure

Although the enamel prisms have been depicted as extending from the junction out to the surface, in practice this is often not the case. Many of the prisms in certain parts of the tooth and in certain teeth stop short of the surface. The surface layers of the tooth are therefore made up of *aprismatic enamel* which may have been produced because the activity of the ameloblasts changes before they cease secretory activity. Too little attention has been paid to this outer layer on the teeth and it is conceivable that it may be related to caries susceptibility and is

certainly of importance when etching and bonding techniques are under consideration.

### Ionic exchange

Once the teeth have erupted, ionic interchange is possible between the crystals of the enamel and ions in the surrounding environment. For example, the calcium ions may be exchanged for strontium and the hydroxyl part of the molecule may be replaced by fluoride which appears to protect the tooth against carious attack. Epidemiological studies have shown that newly erupted teeth may be more susceptible to caries than teeth in more mature individuals, so that great efforts are now made by restorative dentists to prevent so far as possible the commencement of carious attack which will become much less likely in the older individual.

## MORPHOLOGY OF TEETH

The overall shape and detailed morphology of the teeth varies considerably between teeth and even within tooth types. Thus the incisors are quite different in shape to the canines, premolars and molars; and in different individuals premolars may themselves vary somewhat in shape. These factors are also important in restorative dental procedures and should be studied in greater depth in standard texts of tooth morphology.

It is usual in current dental practice to distinguish to some extent between restorative procedures in deciduous teeth and permanent teeth and this is because there are structural differences between them, the most important of which are the relative size of the teeth, the thickness of the enamel and underlying dentine, the relative size of the pulp chambers (which are larger in deciduous teeth) and the bulbosity of the enamel of deciduous teeth at the cervical margin. However, there is evidence accruing recently that the structure of the enamel of deciduous and permanent teeth may differ and this may affect the rate of progression of caries. For instance, it has recently been shown using micro-radiographic techniques that deciduous teeth are less well mineralized than their permanent counterparts. This may account for their whiter appearance, since more porous enamel tends to be less translucent and the yellow of the underlying dentine does not show through so clearly.

## DENTINE STRUCTURE, CHEMISTRY AND SENSITIVITY

### Dentine

The bulk of the structure of the tooth, both crown and root, is made up of a less well mineralized but more flexible tissue known as dentine. This also is composed of hydroxyapatite crystals but in a less concentrated form than in enamel. Most of the crystals are arranged more or less parallel to the enamel–dentine junction but in the three dimensional sense are much more random than those in enamel. They are laid down in a matrix composed of *glycosaminoglycans*, in which have been laid down *collagen fibrils* secreted by the odontoblast cells in their movement inwards from the enamel–dentine junction towards the future pulp. The matrix of dentine therefore consists of a rather dense, rubbery material, the general shape of which is retained even after removal by acids of all of the mineral component. Whilst caries of enamel results in cavitation and loss of the material, at least initially in dentine a rubbery, stained matrix may be retained for some time.

### Odontoblast processes

As the odontoblasts migrate inwards from the junction towards the pulp they leave behind them a cell process which becomes incorporated into the matrix. The dentine is therefore permeated by millions of cell processes radiating out from the odontoblasts, through the whole thickness of the dentine in the younger tooth. These processes may have side communicating branches so that a syncitium of cells is formed. When the dentine mineralizes, crystals are laid down in the matrix and fibres of the matrix but are not laid down in the cell processes. In the mature dentine therefore, the cell processes are contained in mineralized tubules running through the dentine. With increasing age these tubules narrow by the deposition of peritubular dentine and there is still disagreement as to whether mature dentine possesses viable cell processes throughout the length of its tubules.

### Dentinal tubules

Although these tubules radiate from the pulp to the enamel–dentine junction they do not travel in straight lines. In the longitudinal plane they tend to follow a sigmoid curve from the outer dentine towards the pulp so that the cell body is placed more apically than the periphery of the process (Fig. 5.1). This arrangement has some clinical significance which will be discussed later (p. 40).

### Mineralization

Unlike enamel, dentine does not mineralize homogeneously along a mineralization front. There is a delay between laying down the matrix and its mineralization in the form of calcospherites which finally coalesce to produce a more or less homogeneously mineralized tissue. In some parts of the tooth a failure in this fusion of calcospherites seems to occur. Firstly in the coronal portion large non-mineralized, star-shaped spaces are left in many teeth, following an incremental line below the amelodentinal junction. These defects are known as *interglobular spaces* and the cell processes of the odontoblasts run straight through them. Their significance in relation to spread of caries is not known. At the periphery of the root just below the cementum, much smaller defects in mineralization are observed, known as the *granular layer of Tomes*. No clinical significance has been ascribed to this structure.

### Secondary dentine

As the odontoblasts migrate pulpally they lay down the adult form of the tooth, completing the root some two and a half to three and a half years after eruption of the tooth. If they were to continue at this rate of production of dentine then clearly the pulp chamber would be obliterated within a few years of establishment of the dentition. Once the mature outline of the tooth has been completed the odontoblasts slow down and although continuing to migrate inwards do so at a rate enabling the pulp chamber to survive into old age.

The dentine laid down in the initial stages of tooth development is known as *primary dentine* and that laid down after the odontoblasts have slowed is known as *regular secondary dentine*. As we will see in Chapter 6, the odontoblasts may change their rate of production of dentine and its type under the influence of carious attack.

**Dentine sensitivity**

In order to enable dentine to react in this manner to carious attack it must be responsive to outside stimulus and many patients who have suffered cavity preparation under inadequate anaesthesia will testify that this is the case. The exact mechanism is still not clear, largely because technical problems of fixation and examination of tissue remain unsolved. The pulp is well supplied by nerves, both non-medullated (controlling blood vessel tone) and medullated (capable of transmitting common sensation and pain). These latter nerves have endings in a plexus close to the odontoblast cell bodies and also have nerve endings on the cell bodies themselves. There is clear evidence that some of these nerve fibres extend some distance into the dentine and have presumably been incorporated into it during its formation. About 1 in 2000 tubules appear to contain nerve fibres, but only for quite short distances. It is interesting to consider that this so-called sparse innervation is probably greater than that found in the fingertips.

As has been already stated, there is some doubt as to whether living odontoblastic cell processes extend throughout the thickness of the dentine in the mature tooth. If they do, then loss of enamel may result in osmotic changes at the peripheral end of the processes, thus resulting in fluid exchange and distortion of the processes. This event may be transmitted along the process and then converted by transduction into nerve impulses either at the inner third of the processes themselves or at the cell body region. If the cell processes do not extend throughout the thickness of the dentine then it is conceivable that fluid balance changes in the outer part of the tubules may initiate distortion of the processes, eventually resulting in impulses to the nerve plexus.

## ENAMEL–DENTINE JUNCTION

The junction between the enamel and dentine lies on the original basement membrane separating the enamel organ on the outside from the papilla or mesodermal tissue on the inside at an early stage of tooth development. In most human teeth it is not a flat sheet but is deformed into a crater-like appearance producing on section the appearance of scallops. The concavities of these scallops face towards the enamel and the convexities towards the dentine. That is to say the outer surface of the dentine, if the enamel were to be removed, appears like the surface of the moon with irregularly shaped craters. The inner surface of the enamel is composed of convexities fitting into these craters. This has the effect of increasing the surface area between the two tissues. In some parts of the human tooth, particularly near to the neck of the tooth, the enamel–dentine junction may be more or less flat.

## SMEAR LAYER

During restorative procedures, removal of decayed enamel and dentine and extension of the cavity for prevention, retention and access may be carried out using hand instruments, such as chisels and hatchets, but is also commonly done using rotary instruments of various types and speeds. Rotating instruments may result in smearing of the crystal and organic content of both enamel and dentine over the cut surface. This smearing may be a purely physical effect or may be engendered by heat at the point of cutting and grinding. Hand instruments, however sharp, may also cause heavy smearing on the enamel surface, especially on the floor of an approximal box. The clinical implications of the smear layers will be discussed later.

## THE PULP

The pulp and the dentine cannot be separated either anatomically or functionally. Anatomically the cell bodies of the dentinal processes lie in the peripheral region of the pulp and the odontoblast cells in total are therefore intimately associated both with dentine and pulp tissue. Functionally the reaction of both dentine and pulp to external stimuli are dependent upon both the cell processes and bodies of the odontoblasts and therefore reaction is a combined function of both tissues.

The three dimensional shape of the *pulp chamber* varies in different teeth. Thus, in an upper incisor the

Important aspects of basic dental science and clinical restorative dentistry will be emphasized by a few examples.

## Enamel prisms

The reader will have appreciated that the detailed orientation of the enamel prisms is complex, since it varies in different parts of the tooth. In the cuspal region the prisms follow a wavy and complex course, probably adding to the strength of this part of the enamel. In the cervical region they may slope towards the cervical margins, and in deciduous teeth, may be more horizontal in this part of the tooth.

## Surface preparation

It is important that unsupported prisms are not left, since these may be extremely friable. The restorative dentist should seek to ensure that the periphery of the preparation lies along the general direction of the prisms. This produces maximum strength and reduces the likelihood of future fracture at the periphery of the restoration. Clinical practice must be tempered with commonsense, and it is recognized by most restorative dentists that sometimes the load on a particular part of a restoration is minimal and it may not be necessary to follow these guidelines.

The same principles apply to the preparation of the surface of a cavity and attempts are often made to avoid leaving loose enamel crystals present, even though these are invisible to the operator. Thus some operators advocate the cleaning and disinfection of a cavity before placing a restoration. It is probably less important in relation to enamel than to dentine unless bonding techniques are anticipated, in which case the prisms of the enamel must be exposed in order to produce a good key for the resin bond. This latter consideration may be important not only in relation to finishing cavity margins but in preparing surfaces of enamel where bonding to unprepared enamel is required.

## Remineralization

It will be clear from the description of enamel that in biological terms it is a non-healing tissue. This is why most approaches to dental caries in the past have been not so much treatment as repair of an untreatable defect. This is now changing and it is becoming apparent that, at least in the early states of carious attack, demineralization or increased pore spacing in enamel may be repaired to some extent by removing the attacking medium and allowing the super-saturated nature of saliva to take its effect; or, if necessary, by applying super-saturated remineralization solutions to the early carious lesion.

It is now well recognized that caries is not a continuous process but is a start–stop phenomenon. It seems logical to assume, therefore, that the condition in its early stages is reversible; this fact forms the basis for most restorative, preventive and early treatment regimes.

## Saliva and plaque

The importance of saliva and its consequent plaque formation on teeth has already been touched upon. Current opinion holds that removal of plaque by adequate oral hygiene procedures, especially during the first two decades of life, will prevent, or markedly reduce, the prevalence of caries. Extensive restorative procedures are therefore contraindicated in patients unable to control their plaque formation and initially the prevention of caries in children and eventually the management of established caries in adults depends as much upon oral hygiene procedures, diet and fluoride application as upon excellent technical restorative procedures.

## Secondary dentine

Odontoblastic processes in their tubules follow a sigmoid course as they traverse towards the pulp. This is especially the case in the radicular part of the tooth. This means that the cell bodies associated with a particular tubule are much more apically placed than the carious attack at the periphery of the tubule. Any reactive secondary dentine will therefore not be developed directly at the base of the cavity but will be placed more apically. This is an important fact to recognize since the protective effect of secondary dentine in distancing the attack from the pulp is useful in the apical portion of the cavity, but exposure of the pulp is much more likely more cervically.

## Progress of caries

The rate of progression of caries through enamel and

dentine is not known with precision, but it appears to take three to four years for an early lesion to progress through enamel. It is then believed that the rate of progression through dentine is much more rapid. Clinically it is obvious that when the lesion reaches dentine it spreads laterally along the amelodentinal junction and this may be a reflection of the lower mineral content of the dentine and also of the interconnecting lateral processes of the odonto-blastic processes. The importance clinically is that caries has to be followed laterally at the enamel–dentine junction, thereby producing undermined enamel which will need to be subsequently removed.

## Dentine sensitivity

The question of reaction of dentine to external stimuli is one of the most important factors in aiding the dentist in the control of carious attack. We have already noted that progress of caries through dentine is more rapid than through enamel, but this disaster is limited by the fact that the dentine will react to attack, producing ir-regular secondary dentine, sometimes known as tertiary dentine.

Perhaps the interesting question concerning the sensitivity of dentine is not how it is brought about, but why it is necessary in the first place. Sensation in most parts of the body is a defence mechanism, allowing the organism to withdraw from noxious stimuli. A patient cannot readily withdraw the teeth, although they might conceivably seek to place unpleasant foods in another portion of the mouth. It may be that the sensitivity of dentine is concerned more with trophic mechanisms controlling the health of the pulpal tissue and may be associated in some way with the response of the odontoblast and their processes to outside stimuli.

A major difference between dentine and enamel is that the former is capable of responding to carious attack or wear or fracture of the tooth and has a potential for healing. This will be discussed in greater depth in Chapter 6, but the living nature of the odontoblastic processes, cell bodies of the odontoblasts and the continuing ability of the tissue to lay down pre-dentine, mineralizing into dentine, enables the tissue to respond to loss of tooth substance to wall off the vulnerable pulp tissue.

## Pulpal involvement

Some dentinal lesions approaching the pulp may have sterile but cariously affected dentine at their base and a micro-exposure in this region could easily be contaminated from bacteria in the saliva. For this reason it is advisable for the operator to use rubber dam when excavating deep cavities of this nature. If pulpal involvement occurs on a small scale the tooth should be made caries free at the enamel–dentine junction, and in a symptomless tooth calcium hydroxide can be used as an indirect pulp capping agent which will encourage the laying down of reparative dentine walling off the lesion. If there is frank exposure of the pulp with bacterial invasion then eventually endodontic treatment will be necessary, but, in the short term and to produce comfort for the patient, anti-inflammatory drugs may be placed over the carious exposure. It is very important in the initial stages of treatment planning to investigate all teeth with carious lesions and to excavate active caries and to dress temporarily the cavities by one or other of these methods. This not only allows the patient to remain in comfort whilst a lengthy treatment plan is carried out, but also allows the teeth to respond to sedative dressings, thereby making future cavity preparation less hazardous.

Because of the sigmoid nature of the dentinal tubules, particularly in the root, the response to stimuli will be more apically placed than the stimulus itself and this should be remembered during cavity preparation because the gingival base of the cavity will be better protected than the coronal portion which is more easily exposed into the pulp.

## Bonding to dentine

Etching and bonding of restorative materials to dentine may be much more difficult than to enamel but the glass-ionomer cements being tooth coloured restorative materials were amongst the first to adhere both to enamel and to dentine. There is scope for much more research in this area, but at the present time cements of this nature may be the treatment of choice for root caries where the production of retentive cavities may be extremely difficult.

# 6. Pathology of caries and pulpal disorders

*D. K. Whittaker*

Caries is essentially an attack on the mineralized tissues of the body, resulting in demineralization and in some cases in destruction of the matrix. In principle it may occur in all of the hard tissues, including bone, but discussion here will be restricted largely to enamel and dentine. In the young, healthy human the dentine of the tooth is entirely protected by enamel or by the gingivae and periodontal tissues in the root area. Caries must therefore commence at the enamel surface. In older individuals where gingival recession and loss of periodontal and bone support has occurred the root of the tooth may be exposed to the mouth and caries may then occur de novo on the cementum and dentine.

## FACTORS INFLUENCING CARIES

The crown of the tooth is in a micro-environment of its own, mainly that of the saliva, microbial deposits derived from the saliva and other sources, food debris and other dietary constituents. Whether caries commences or not seems to depend upon the quality of this environment, the ability of the tooth to resist demineralization, immunological reactions by the host and the length of time for which all these factors are in operation. The disease therefore has been described as *multifactorial* and in some texts as many as 50 factors have been described in relation to carious attack. It is more profitable to group the factors into three. First, those associated with the host, including the quality of the saliva and the bacterial flora therein. Secondly, outside factors associated with diet and the substrate on which these bacteria act and, finally, the tooth itself and those features which either predispose to or resist carious attack (Fig. 6.1).

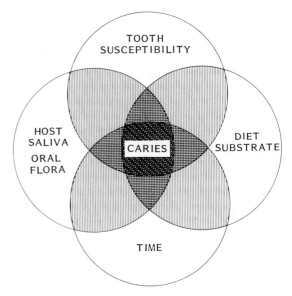

**Fig. 6.1** Factors influencing the onset and spread of dental caries. Microbial breakdown products of dietary components may produce an adverse local environment which, if operative for sufficient time, may result in caries in a susceptible tooth.

## Host factors

When a tooth is developing within the alveolar process its enamel surface is protected by means of an *organic pellicle* and cellular covering. As it erupts into the oral cavity much of this protection is lost, but immediately on contact with the saliva a secondary organic pellicle is laid down on the enamel surface; it is to this that organisms within the oral cavity attach themselves.

### Micro-organisms

Initially, most of the organisms are streptococcal in nature, producing an immature plaque on the surface of the tooth. If this is allowed to be maintained other organisms of filamentous nature, such as *Actinomyces* will also be involved and the plaque is said to be mature. The organisms colonizing the plaque will depend upon those present in the oral cavity and may therefore vary from individual to individual. However, it has recently been shown that breast-fed children may acquire *Streptococcus mutans* from their mother so that, in this sense, caries may be thought of as an infectious disease.

There has been a great deal of research to establish the nature of organisms associated with dental caries, much of which lies outside the scope of this chapter. Some of this work has been carried out on gnotobiotic animals, where it was shown that the difference between animals which were caries active and those which were caries resistant lay in the fact that the latter lacked particular microorganisms. In human enamel caries large numbers of organisms have been described on the enamel surface, but in caries susceptible individuals it seems that the most obvious organisms are *Lactobacilli* and *Streptococcus mutans*. In older plaques, *Actinomyces* species are present, but most studies have not especially implicated these in the development of the early lesion. In the case of root caries the most commonly isolated organisms are of the *Actinomyces* type, followed by *Lactobacilli*, *Streptococcus mutans* and *Streptococcus sanguis*.

## Saliva

Not only is the saliva responsible for the micro-environment of plaque organisms but is also in itself important in the development of early carious lesions. This is because caries is essentially a demineralizing disease requiring a fall in pH at the surface of the tooth. If the saliva is capable of resisting this change in pH because of *buffering capacity* then caries is less likely to ensue. It is known that high flow rates of saliva improve its buffering capacity so that caries is dependent not only on the quality of the saliva but also upon its quantity. It is for instance well known that caries increases in patients with xerostomia following irradiation of tumours in the oral region, but there may also be changes of diet associated with these problems. Saliva is a super-saturated solution of calcium, phosphate, hydroxyl and fluoride ions; these may reduce the solubility of

enamel and promote remineralization of early lesions. In addition, the saliva contains non-specific antibacterial agents (such as lysozyme, lacto-peroxidase and lactoferin) and immunoglobulin IgA molecules and, in those patients with inflammation of the periodontal tissues, IgG may be present in the serum exudate. It has been suggested that it may be possible to immunize patients against caries but in western society where caries prevalence appears to be falling it seems unlikely that this will be an acceptable procedure.

## Oral hygiene

The final host factor of importance in caries is the ability to improve oral hygiene, thereby removing the plaque from the surface of the teeth and preventing the production of acids initiating caries. Oral hygiene is usually considered to be mechanical, using toothbrushes, toothpastes, floss and similar methods, but it must be remembered that oral hygiene is also a natural phenomenon which some individuals do well and others do not. The use of the tongue as a means of oral hygiene has received relatively little study but may well be a factor in reducing caries.

## Diet

The second main group of factors associated with caries of the teeth is that of diet. Microbial plaque on the surface of teeth is only disastrous if there is sufficient substrate for these bacteria to work upon. Fermentable carbohydrates needs to be present for acid to be formed. The problem is that in the presence of fermentable carbohydrates, the plaque bacteria produce acid rapidly so that the pH in relation to the plaque falls very quickly. The recovery from this position to normal pH levels is an extended process. The major part of our dietary fermentable carbohydrate is sucrose, but lactose is present in milk, and maltose is derived from the hydrolysis of starch. It seems that it is the frequency of fall in pH which is important and this information enables dentists to plan dietary advice for their patients. Attempts have been made to replace these fermentable carbohydrates with other types of sugar such as xylitol which is a sugar alcohol but is not metabolized to acid by the plaque organisms. There are, however, difficulties in changing the dietary habits of a lifetime.

## Tooth susceptibility

The third factor related to caries incidence appears to be the structure of the teeth themselves.

### Morphology

Caries tends to occur at certain points on the teeth, such as the depth of the fissures and below the contact areas and cervical margins, and this suggests that the shape and morphology of the tooth is important along with its ability or otherwise to shed food debris or to be cleansed by the patient's musculature or salivary flow. Packing of food between teeth which are malaligned may also constitute a problem. Fissures which are deep and difficult to cleanse may well be more liable to caries than shallow, cleanable fissures; the details of tooth morphology are best studied in texts related to that subject.

### Chemistry

Using techniques of microprobe analysis and micro-biopsy it has been possible to show that teeth structure varies chemically between different individuals. For example fluoride levels vary between individuals and this in itself may have an influence on their caries resistance.

### Surface structure

It has become clear that the outer surface structure of enamel is extremely variable, and indeed in many patients in some of their teeth and at certain sites the prisms of the enamel may in fact not reach the surface. The surface of the tooth in contact with the micro-environment is therefore said to be *aprismatic*, but the relationship of this structural variation to caries resistance is not clear.

## RESEARCH METHODS

Most of the modern techniques of scientific investigation have been applied to caries over the decades. These have included epidemiological studies on the incidence of the disease and biochemical studies on the environment of the mouth and of the teeth themselves. It is beyond the scope of this book to discuss these in any detail. However, in order to understand the principles of restorative dentistry, it is necessary to have a working knowledge of the pathology of the lesion itself.

## Ground sections in polarized light

Most of the early work in this area consisted of the production of ground sections through teeth containing natural early lesions and much of it was directed towards the technology of producing sufficiently thin sections to be of use in these studies. Sections of between 50 and 100 $\mu$m have now been achieved and these may be examined either with the light microscope or, more profitably and commonly, with the polarized light microscope.

*Polarized light* vibrates in one plane, and this plane may be rotated by suitable crystalline materials. Enamel is such a material, as is dentine by nature of its hydroxyapatite content and its collagen matrix. When polarized light is passed through enamel it is rotated both by the crystals themselves and by the arrangement of the crystals in the form of prisms. The former is said to be intrinsic birefringence and the latter, form birefringence. In the case of dentine the light is rotated by the crystals of hydroxyapatite and also by the repeat pattern of the collagen. Carious attack affects both the size and shape of the crystals and the spaces between them and the overall outline of the enamel prisms. In the case of dentine it may alter the collagen component as well. For these reasons carious lesions exhibit altered birefringence, the direction and extent of which not only indicates the extent of the lesion but may be used quantitatively to deduce the degree of demineralization.

## Transmission electron microscopy

The availability of the transmission electron microscope (TEM) in the early 1960s held promise of detailed investigation both of normal and carious enamel, but it proved almost impossible to produce sections of sufficient thinness for this technique to be fully exploited. Thin sectioning is possible in partially demineralized enamel but there is the possibility that the sectioning procedure may alter the crystalline structure of the material being examined. Attempts were made to solve this problem by cutting thick sections through the lesions and taking carbon replicas, which themselves could be examined in the TEM; considerable progress was made using this technique.

## Scanning electron microscopy

A decade later, the scanning electron microscope (SEM) became available and, since this records information from a cut surface by excitation of secondary electrons, thin sectioning was no longer needed. Although the method has been exploited to some extent in studies of caries, interpretation of the images and particularly the formation of smear layers during sectioning has proved difficult. Methods of removal of the smear layer using either chemical or, preferably, ion etching techniques are now in progress and back scatter electron imaging, which provides information from beneath the cut surface, is a recent promising advance. Modern SEMs allow analysis of X-rays emitted from the specimen being studied, and electron microprobe analysis of this nature allows chemical analysis to be made in various parts of the lesion. X-ray and electron crystallography have also featured in studies of caries.

## Microradiography

Since carious lesions in both enamel and dentine are characterized by loss of mineral, microradiographs can be used to demonstrate changes of mineral density within the lesions. It is necessary to use a graduated step wedge in order that a standard may be compared with the radiographic image and plano-parallel sections of known thickness are required in order to make the necessary calculations of mineral loss.

## Microbiopsy

Recently microbiopsy techniques have been developed so that small portions of a carious lesion from a known position can be excised and analysed using some of the methods previously described but are also available for biochemical study. Using such techniques the distribution for instance of fluoride ions within a lesion may be determined.

All of these methods have now been applied both to natural human lesions and to artificially induced lesions in human and in animal teeth, so that the process of caries in mineralized tissues is now more fully, but still incompletely, understood.

## CARIES OF ENAMEL

When mineral is removed from the enamel by carious attack, the individual crystals making up the prisms diminish in size and the enamel is said to become more porous.

## The white spot lesion

Even a slight increase in porosity of the enamel changes its optical characteristics and in the initial stages it becomes less translucent so that the earliest evidence of caries is known as a white spot lesion. At this stage the surface of the enamel is still intact and the lesion may be difficult to detect clinically. Histological studies using polarized light have shown that the lesion at this stage is not continuously progressive but may *remineralize* so that processes of both destruction and repair are occurring simultaneously. When examined under the polarizing microscope in water, the lesion is described as cone shaped with its base just below an intact surface zone. The body of the lesion appears to be dark in colour and the incremental lines are accentuated. The use of quinoline as an inhibition medium of different refractive index allows further details of the early lesion to be described. Four zones may be seen in an early white spot lesion (Fig. 6.2).

### Advancing front

Zone 1 is a translucent zone present at the advancing front of the lesion and is usually only seen in sections examined in quinoline. This zone is more porous than sound enamel, having a pore volume of about 1% compared with 0.1% in intact enamel.

### Dark zone

Zone 2 is known as the dark zone and lies superficial to the translucent zone. It appears dark when

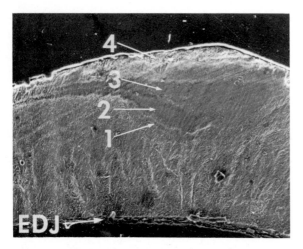

**Fig. 6.2** Scanning electron micrograph of a ground section of an early 'white spot' carious lesion. It consists of four zones: 1, Translucent; 2, Dark zone; 3, Body of the lesion; 4, Surface zone. EDJ, Enamel–dentine junction.

examined in quinoline. Polarized light studies have shown that the pore volume is increased to 2–4% in this region. It is thought that the dark appearance is occasioned because some of the pores are too small to allow quinoline to enter so that they retain air following sectioning. It has been speculated that some remineralization may be occurring here, reducing some of the pore sizes.

*Lesion body*

Zone 3 is the body of the lesion and since more than 5% of the enamel is porous and the size of the pores are large enough to allow water to enter, the body appears dark when examined under polarized light in water, but translucent when examined in quinoline. In some parts of the body the pore volume may increase to 25%.

*Surface zone*

Zone 4 is known as the surface zone and is best seen in sections examined in water. It is an intact surface layer with a pore volume of less than 1% and is usually 20–50 $\mu$m in thickness. Thus, the early lesion is more demineralized in its depth than at its surface and although it was first thought that the surface zone was caused by a hypermineralized zone at the

surface of the tooth, it may be reproduced following removal of this surface layer. It is now thought that it may be caused by recrystallization of dissolved mineral elements from deeper in the lesion.

### Fissure caries

The foregoing description is that of an early lesion on the smooth surface of a tooth and in the case of early fissure caries similar appearances are seen around the fissure wall. It should be noted that in many fissures examined in sections there is an enamel defect at the base so that the lesion spreads very quickly into dentine. This may explain the recently described phenomenon of 'bomb' caries in teeth that have been subjected to fluoride ions during development or subsequently. The enamel around the sides of the fissure is resistant to carious attack by reason of its fluoride content but the lesion spreads rapidly into dentine spreading along the enamel–dentine junction and cavitating the dentine although the fissure may appear clinically to be intact.

### Electron microscopy

Electron microscope studies on early carious lesions have provided conflicting evidence. In most cases the inter-prismatic regions seem to be preferentially dissolved but also larger, unusually shaped crystals may be seen in this region and these may represent a remineralization phenomenon. The biopsy techniques previously described have shown that in the translucent zone the cross-section diameter of the crystals is 25–30 nm compared with 30–40 nm in sound enamel. In the dark zone of the lesion, crystal diameters may be 50–100 nm, whereas in the main body of the lesion they may be only 10 nm in diameter. These findings again support the view that remineralization of crystals is occurring in various parts of the early carious lesion.

### Microradiography

Microradiographs of sections through the early lesion are sufficiently sensitive to demonstrate loss of mineral if this is more than about 5%. The body of the lesion therefore shows up well using this technique and the intact surface zone is also readily seen. In high resolution microradiography the outline of the incremental lines may be visible within the body of the lesion.

Biochemical studies using biopsies of the lesion or electron probe micro-analysis have confirmed these changes in enamel caries and have also shown that fluoride levels are high in this artificially porous material.

### Progress of the lesion

As the lesion progresses through the enamel its apex may reach the enamel–dentine junction before collapse of the intact surface zone occurs, so that lesions may be quite deep before they are easily detectable clinically. The enamel lesion, however, is extremely porous by this stage, so that acids are able to diffuse easily across the junction and into the dentine. The implication is that dentine may be involved even when lesions appear to be restricted to enamel on standard clinical radiographs.

## CARIES IN DENTINE

Caries spreading to dentine may be either subsequent to enamel caries having reached the enamel–dentine junction or in certain circumstances, such as exposure of the root of the tooth, it may commence de novo in the cementum and spread to the dentine directly.

### Coronal caries

Involvement of dentine in the crown of the tooth may be either underneath smooth surface enamel caries, usually at the contact area or immediately below it, or may be an extension of caries in an occlusal fissure. When the carious process reaches the enamel–dentine junction, it tends to spread laterally involving the dentine on a wider front. In this way the enamel is undermined so that the resultant cavity preparation requires removal of sound enamel in order that the infected dentine may be approached and also removal of unsupported enamel prisms, which will tend to fracture under stress. Lesions of the occlusal fissures may directly involve dentine, since in many cases enamel is deficient at the base of the fissure.

### Root caries

In patients whose root surfaces have become exposed, usually due to chronic inflammatory periodontal disease, but also due to continuing eruption to compensate for occlusal wear, the root becomes directly exposed to plaque and carious attack. Chronic infective periodontal disease and continuing eruption due to occlusal wear are both commonly seen in older people, hence root caries tends to be a disease of old age. Root caries may extend from lesions at the cervical margin of the enamel or may attack dentine exposed directly by the aforementioned means. Root caries can be of two types: active root caries is soft and pale in colour, whereas arrested lesions, possibly caused by good oral hygiene techniques, tend to stain and be hard and dark brown.

Dentine is a living reactive tissue and must be considered in association with the living pulp tissue beneath. Reactions to dentine caries therefore involve consideration of both the dentine itself and the underlying pulp tissue. The reaction and response of the pulp will be considered later.

### Microorganisms

Once the enamel has been penetrated bacteria can gain access directly to the dentinal tubules and so the tissue becomes infected. The initial invasion of dentine appears to be mainly acidogenic, the acid presumably diffusing ahead of any microorganisms. The first organisms to invade the dentine appear to be *Lactobacilli* and also cariogenic *Streptococci*, notably *Streptococcus mutans*. Underneath the enamel–dentine junction the microbiological population is mixed and organisms producing proteolytic hydrolytic enzymes may be found. At the advancing edge of the dentinal lesion is a zone of demineralized dentine which bacteria have not yet penetrated. This is because the tubules are smaller than the diameter of most bacteria and only when the tubules have become laterally enlarged by dissolution of the intertubular matrix do bacteria enter. Superficial to the demineralized dentine is a zone of penetration in which bacteria are present in the tubules. Superficial to that again is a zone of complete destruction where the mineral content and organic matrix of the dentine have both been destroyed.

## Effect on dentinal tubules

Once the dentine is infected it may react in several different ways. Those tubules located in the centre of the demineralized zone may appear to be empty because the cell processes of the odontoblasts have withdrawn. During section preparation these empty tubules may be filled with air, producing a dark colour under the light microscope often referred to as a dead tract.

Odontoblastic cell processes less acutely involved in the carious process, that is, usually those at the periphery of the lesion may react by laying down calcified material as the cell processes withdraw, thereby equalizing the refractive index of the dentine and producing a transparent or translucent sclerotic zone. The crystals in these tubules, when examined in the electron microscope may have larger and more irregular crystals than in the normal dentine. They are considered to represent the result of remineralization. Sclerotic dentine may be considered as an extension of the normal process of production of peritubular dentine. The sclerotic dentine may consist initially of fine crystals of whitlockite and, at later stages of mineralization, of a mixture of whitlockite and hydroxyapatite. The final obliteration of the tubule appears to be by hydroxyapatite crystals.

## Secondary and tertiary dentine

The lesion eventually spreads towards the pulp of the tooth and the stimulus may cause reactionary tertiary dentine to be laid down in the pulp at the depth of the lesion in an attempt to wall off the advancing caries from the pulp. It may be a relatively well formed tissue containing dentinal tubules and may be similar in structure to normal secondary dentine; or it may be an abnormal tissue with very few tubules and numerous interglobular zones. Reactionary dentine is most frequently formed when the stimulus is mild and the blood supply to the pulp is good, so it is more likely to be seen in younger teeth. If the stimulus is overwhelming, the odontoblast cells lining the pulp may be killed and then of course no reactionary dentine can be produced. Under these circumstances the carious lesion will directly involve the pulp; this will be discussed in the next section.

## THE RESPONSE OF THE PULP

In the early stages of infection, the pulp reacts as would any other healthy tissue.

## Hyperaemia

An inflammatory reaction occurs and in its initial stages this is characterized by hyperaemia. The pulpal blood vessels dilate, become more permeable and fluid and defence cells pass out into the surrounding pulp tissue. This increases the pressure within the pulp and this pressure, unlike in soft tissues, cannot be relieved because of the enclosed nature of the pulpal tissue. The pressure therefore rises and the patient suffers pain. Initially this may be the case when transient stimuli such as very hot or very cold liquids are placed in contact with a carious lesion. The pain may only last as long as the stimulus is applied. Once the carious lesion has approached closely to the pulp the stimulus may be continuous and the reaction of the pulp will depend upon the duration and the intensity of this stimulus.

## Chronic inflammation

If the lesion is progressing slowly towards the pulp then toxins and thermal stimulation may be of a low grade nature and the result is chronic inflammation. Lymphocytes, plasma cells, macrophages and monocytes can be seen in the pulpal tissue and the tissue may survive.

## Acute inflammation

If the stimuli reaching the pulp are stronger, then the blood vessels dilate, fluid passes out into the tissues and the pressure builds up to such an extent that the arterioles entering through the apical foramina may be occluded. Polymorphonuclear leucocytes are the main cells involved in acute inflammation.

## Periapical involvement

Eventually the inflammation will spread out of the pulp chamber through the apical foramina to the periapical tissues. The response of these tissues may also be either acute or chronic, depending upon the severity of the stimulus. Similar events within the pulp may occur in caries of the roots of the teeth, depending again upon the severity of the onslaught.

## RELATIONSHIP TO CLINICAL MANAGEMENT

It should be clear from this description of the pathology of the carious lesion that in its earliest stages, i.e. the white spot lesion, there may be considerable difficulties in clinical diagnosis.

### Early caries

The surface of the enamel will still be intact and therefore the lesions can only be diagnosed either visually or radiographically. The use of a mirror and strong lighting may indicate a slight change in optical density below the contact area and high intensity transillumination with a small fibreoptic probe may be more useful. Bitewing radiographs are unlikely to pick up the very early lesion and it is said that by the time a lesion is visible using this means it may well have progressed towards the enamel–dentine junction. All is not lost however, since changes in oral hygiene practice, removal of plaque, administration of fluorides and good dietary control may cause such lesions to remineralize even though they were never diagnosed.

### Remineralization

Since these early lesions are cycling between destruction and repair, the clinician aims to tip the balance towards repair. There is some evidence that such remineralized lesions may resist further attack better than normal enamel. It may be that many patients diagnosed as caries-free, have in fact remineralized early lesions from their own saliva.

Once cavitation of the surface has occurred, remineralization will not replace the normal contour of the tooth. For this reason probing should not be used in diagnosis of early lesions, since cavitation may be produced by the clinician. The early diagnosis of carious lesions has been discussed in Chapter 2.

Very early caries is perhaps best diagnosed by a study of the risk factors to which the patient is subjected. Therefore, a good dietary history will be needed and it is clear that the younger patient is at greater risk than the older. The adequate secretion of saliva and its buffering capacity should be investigated and it may be useful to look at the types of organisms present in the saliva so that the high risk *Lactobacilli* and *Strep. mutans* may be discerned.

### Excavation of caries

Once the caries has involved the dentine it will be necessary to remove softened and infected necrotic material. It is clear from the progression of the lesion that this may involve a larger cavity than at first appreciated since the lesion will have extended along the enamel–dentine junction. It is currently believed necessary to remove all of the infected dentine at the junction. When the softened dentine in the bulk of the lesion has been removed the decision has to be made on how to deal with the infected area of dentine overlying the pulp. A current approach is to excavate the infected dentine leaving the attacked translucent zone over the pulp intact. The determination of this zone has largely relied on clinical experience but recently dyes have been produced which may stain the infected dentine but not the translucent zone (Ch. 10). Providing the tooth has been symptomless and appears to be vital the translucent area of dentine covering the pulp may be capped with a calcium hydroxide paste, the rationale here being to protect the pulp and induce the formation of reparative dentine. If there is clinical evidence of acute or chronic inflammation of the pulp, usually by symptoms, then the inevitable sequel may be death of the pulp, requiring eventual root canal therapy. Decisions as to how to stabilize and treat the initial carious lesions should be made in the early appointments before planning the detailed restorative treatment. Thus it is far better to treat temporarily all the lesions in the mouth at an early stage rather than going ahead with definitive restorative treatment of a few.

The reactions of the pulp underlying carious lesions may give some clinical information to the dentist as to the health or otherwise of the tissues. Thus, a patient who complains of transient pain following hot and cold drinks, the pain lasting for the duration of the stimulus, may well have pulpal hyperaemia which may be reversible if stabilization of the cavity is achieved using the methods described. Once the pulp has become infected it may, if the inflammation is chronic, produce no symptoms. Under these circumstances the patient may have no pain and the pulp may eventually recover. However, it may slowly die without symptoms and the dentist should be aware of this possibility and keep future checks on the health and vitality of that particular tooth. If the patient complains of continuous lancing pain then the tooth pulp is almost certainly acutely inflamed and a vital removal of the pulp or the tooth is probably indicated. In patients where this has not occurred the acute continuous pain may eventually resolve for a time as the inflammation expands through the apical foramen and the pressure is released. During hyperaemia the patient may be able to localize the intermittent sharp pain to a particular tooth but when acute pulpitis intervenes the pain may radiate over a larger area. As the inflammation extends into the periapical tissues, and in the absence of the satisfactory response by the patient, it may eventually involve alveolar bone. The pain then may become deep-seated and throbbing and may be localizable because the tooth is tender to percussion or biting. If the infection extends to the bone, producing a localized osteomyelitis, it may then track through the bone, reducing the pressure and therefore the pain but then raise the periosteum either buccally or lingually to produce severe pain again and cause an apical abscess. If this abscess discharges into the buccal or lingual sulci the pain may again cease because of reduction of pressure. However, it may spread above the level of attachment of the muscles of the mandible and maxilla and the final sequel is a cellulitis or facial swelling over the area. Patients are likely to seek emergency dental treatment at any point where the pressure is high either in the pulp, the periapical tissues, the bone or the facial tissues. Reduction of pressure at certain stages of the advance of the infection explains why patients frequently sit in the dental chair saying: 'The pain was acute but it stopped as soon as I came to see the dentist'.

# 7. Functional anatomy of the occlusion

*D. K. Whittaker   P. H. Jacobsen*

Whilst the word 'occlusion' strictly refers to the act of closing the teeth together, it has come to mean the way in which the teeth are aligned in each jaw, and how they contact each other and those of the opposing arch during the complicated movements of chewing or speaking. The concept has inevitably also come to include the way in which the mandible moves in relation to the skull. The study of occlusion in a functional sense therefore includes the temporo-mandibular joints and their neuro-muscular control, as well as the teeth themselves.

The masticatory apparatus is unique in the whole body because of the close interactions between differing structural entities. Malfunctions in the joints themselves, the muscles operating them, the neuro-muscular reflexes controlling them or imperfections in the interdigitation of up to 32 teeth may all result in dysfunction of the masticatory apparatus as a whole.

## THE TEMPOROMANDIBULAR JOINTS

The articulation between the fused right and left portions of the maxilla and mandible is by the temporomandibular joints (TMJ). Each is unique in the body in terms of function since it is the only place in which left and right joints are linked via a relatively inflexible bone, the mandible. This means that movements of each joint may not take place independently of the other, and therefore it is possible that undue stresses on one joint may be transmitted to the other. The joints are also unique in that their pattern of movement and the forces transmitted to them are modified by the teeth.

## Anatomy

The upper part of the TMJ is composed of the *glenoid fossa* which is an oval depression in the base of the temporal bone. This depression is bounded anteriorly by the *articular eminence*, a bony swelling down which the head of the *mandibular condyle* will move during function.

The glenoid fossa lies immediately in front of the external auditory meatus, and its posterior border is limited by the squamo-tympanic fissure and the post-glenoid tubercle. The tubercle is a small, conical eminence separating the articular surface from the anterior margin of the tympanic part of the bone. The roof of the glenoid fossa is sufficiently thin to be transparent if transilluminated in a dried skull, which suggests that the joint is not adapted to bear much stress.

The other half of the joint is the *condylar process* of the mandible, a rounded structure about 15–20 mm in the mesiolateral dimension and 8–10 mm antero-posteriorly. The long axis of each condyle is angulated so that lines drawn through them will meet at a point posterior to the mandible itself. This is because the condyles appear to be set at right angles to the line of the molar teeth on each side.

In the adult, the articulating bony surfaces of both condyle and glenoid fossa are composed of dense cortical bone which is covered by dense fibrous connective tissue.

### Ligaments

The ligaments probably do not support the joint during normal function, but restrict the *border movements* of the mandible, and therefore define the *envelope* within which all movements occur. There are four ligaments associated with the joint.

The *temporomandibular ligament* extends from the base of the zygomatic process of the temporal bone and the articular tubercle, and runs downwards and backwards to be inserted into the neck of the condyle. It appears to be separate from, and lateral to, the *capsular ligament*, which forms a kind of collar around the neck of the condyle and runs upwards to be attached around the periphery of the glenoid fossa. The capsular ligament completely surrounds the joint cavity to form a synovial capsule. During opening of the jaw, the temporomandibular ligament restricts hinge movement, but when wider opening occurs, the head of the condyle moves forward onto the articular eminence, which relaxes the temporomandibular ligament, and causes the third ligament, the *sphenomandibular*, to become taut. This ligament is situated some distance from the joint itself, and arises from the spinous process of the sphenoid bone, passing downwards and forwards to be inserted into the lingula on the lingual side of the ramus of the mandible. The fourth ligament is the *stylomandibular*, which extends from the styloid process to the posterior border of the angle.

### The temporomandibular disc

The joint cavity is divided into upper and lower compartments by a biconcave, oval shaped disc of fibrous tissue which is sandwiched between the head of the condyle and the bone of the glenoid fossa. Its inferior surface is concave and its superior surface convex, and it has the appearance of a baseball cap placed over the head of the condyle with the peak arranged anteriorly.

The crown of the cap is thickened by a posterior band of dense connective tissue, and, at the junction of the crown and the peak of the cap, there is a second thickening, the anterior fibrous band. Between these bands is a less dense intermediate zone, and behind the posterior band is the bilaminar region, consisting of an upper part attached to the posterior wall of the glenoid fossa and a lower part attached to the back of the condyle (Fig. 7.1).

The borders of the disc are attached to the fibrous capsule of the joint, except anteriorly, where the peak of the disc is attached to fibres of the lateral

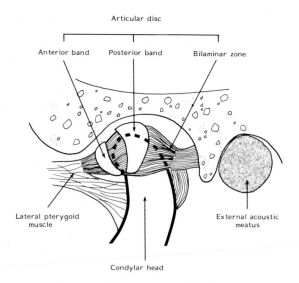

**Fig. 7.1** Anatomy of the temporomandibular joint, showing the articular disc (meniscus) as the shape of a baseball cap lying over the condylar head, and dividing the joint space into upper and lower compartments.

pterygoid muscle. There may be some attachment of the disc laterally to fibres of the masseter and temporal muscles. Posteriorly, the disc is attached to a thick layer of vascularized connective tissue, and in this region the disc contains elastic fibres. The part of the capsule inserted into the disc from above, which is that attached to the glenoid fossa, is loose and therefore permits extensive sliding movements of the upper joint compartment.

The lower part of the capsule, which attaches the disc to the neck of the condyle, is much denser, allowing only hinge movement in the lower joint compartment. A synovial membrane, composed of connective tissue with many capillaries, lines the peripheral parts of the disc and the capsule. It secretes synovial fluid into the joint spaces which has a jelly-like consistency and is composed largely of hyaluronic acid. The amount of synovial fluid present in normal function is very small and it is assumed that the joint spaces are normally collapsed.

### Microscopic anatomy of the joint

**The bones.** The articular surfaces consist of fibrous connective tissue overlying undifferentiated mesoderm, which itself overlies a thin layer of hyaline cartilage. This cartilage is more predominant in younger joints, and is a growth cartilage taking part in the normal development of the joint, and may be involved in remodelling processes in adulthood.

Below the layer of cartilage is compact bone covering the cancellous bone of the internal structure of the mandible. In old age, not only may the cartilage zone be lost, but so may the fibrous tissue covering at least some areas, resulting in denuding of the compact bone layer.

***The disc.*** The central part of the disc consists of dense connective tissue, but peripherally it has a looser texture, rich in vessels and nerves, particularly posteriorly in the bilaminar region. The capsule and parts of the disc are innervated by branches of the auriculo-temporal nerve, which are arranged so that they are not compressed during movements of the joint.

The blood supply to the TMJ is from the superficial branch of the external carotid artery.

## TEMPOROMANDIBULAR JOINT FUNCTION

From the clinical viewpoint, understanding the occlusion depends in the first instance upon understanding the large number of definitions that relate to it.

As was described above, the TMJ is capable of two movements — rotation and sliding (translation).

Rotation occurs in the lower compartment and sliding in the upper. The disc should locate on the head of the condyle throughout, though during sliding it lags behind the condyle somewhat, so that the condyle comes to bear on the anterior fibrous thickening. During the return movement, the elasticity of the bilaminar zone moves the disc back.

If the disc gets out of phase or looses its elasticity, then 'clicks' occur during movement as the fibrous tissue relocates on the condylar head.

Lateral movement of the condyles within the fossae occurs as the mandible moves to the left or right and is called *side shift*.

The medial pole of each condyle is well located in its glenoid fossa medially, and this is what determines the axis about which it turns; the *hinge axis*. There is a *true* hinge axis, i.e. the real one, and an *arbitrary* hinge axis, derived for use with articulators (Ch. 12).

The *terminal hinge axis* is coincident with *centric relation* (CR) at the correct *vertical dimension*.

CR is a position of the condyle within the glenoid fossa unrelated to tooth position and several definitions exist for it. That used most in the UK is, 'the most retruded position of the condyle from which unstrained lateral movements are possible'. But, 'the most superior, posterior position' is a rather better definition for practical, clinical use.

When the mandible moves to open the mouth, it will initially describe an arc about the terminal hinge

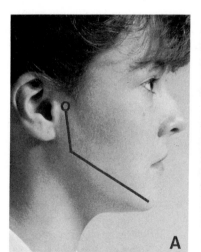 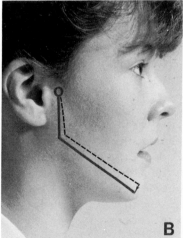 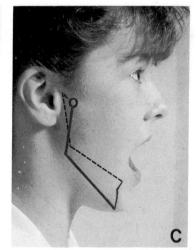

**Fig. 7.2** Opening the mouth from the retruded contact position (A), the mandible first describes an arc on the terminal hinge axis (B), followed by protrusion and rotation to wide opening (C). This movement is the posterior border of Posselt's envelope. Opening from centric occlusion would trace an arc slightly anterior to this.

axis. At about 15 mm open, further hinge movement is impossible, and the condyles slide forwards, taking their discs with them, and continue the rotation on a wider arc until maximum opening is reached (Fig. 7.2). The pathway described forms the posterior boundary of the *envelope* of border movements. As was described earlier, the envelope is determined to a large extent by the ligaments around the TMJ.

## THE MUSCLES OF MASTICATION

These may be divided simplistically into closing and opening muscles. However, it must be remembered that relaxation of the closing muscles is necessary to allow the opening muscles to operate, so that all the muscles are operational during mandibular movement.

The *masseter* is made up of two main bundles of muscle fibres extending from the lower border of the zygomatic arch, downwards and slightly backwards, to be inserted on the lateral side of the ramus of the mandible. Its major function is to close the jaws together with great force, although it may also protrude the mandible slightly during this movement.

The *temporal* muscle is broadly inserted over the lateral surface of the parietal bone and its anterior fibres run more or less vertically, its middle fibres obliquely, and its posterior fibres almost horizontally, all to be inserted into the coronoid process. It is used to position the mandible during closing movements. Usually, the anterior fibres contract first, elevating the mandible, followed by the others to control fine positioning. The activity of the temporal muscle is extremely complex and unilateral contraction is involved in lateral mandibular excursions. The muscle is extremely important in dysfunction (Ch. 20), since the pain arising from its spasm is reported by patients as headache.

The *masseter* is made up of two main bundles of pterygoid fossa and its fibres run downwards, backwards and outwards to be inserted into the inner aspect of the ramus. It is able to elevate the mandible and position it laterally. During protrusive and lateral movements, the activity of this muscle is greater than that of the temporals.

The *lateral pterygoid* muscle has two heads, one arising from the outer part of the lateral pterygoid plate and the other from the base of the sphenoid bone. The two heads come together and are inserted into both the neck of the condyle, and through the anterior wall of the capsule into the disc. The main function of this muscle is to draw both the head of the condyle and the disc forwards during opening movements. Unilateral contraction will produce lateral movement of the mandible in association with the other muscles.

There are *minor muscles of mastication* which include the *digastric* and the *buccinator*. The digastric is an opening muscle running from the mastoid process to a bursa on the hyoid bone and up to the genial tubercles of the mandible. Contraction will draw the chin downwards, but this is aided considerably by gravity so that the muscle is most prominent in the final opening movements. The buccinator muscles are concerned with maintaining the muscular activity of the cheeks and retaining food on the occlusal planes of the teeth.

## THE TEETH

### Centric occlusion

Centric occlusion (CO) is the position of maximum intercuspation of the teeth and, when articulating models, is usually the position where exact interdigitation occurs — the 'best fit'.

CO is the major reference position for occlusal restoration; the vast majority of restorations are adjusted with the patient moving to maximum intercuspation. The condylar position in CO is 1–2 mm anterior to centric relation, and this discrepancy appears to be physiologically necessary, though the reason is unknown.

When CO has been lost, in full dentures for instance, or is unsatisfactory, CR has to be found as the reference position. Then the new CO is made with the condyles in CR, though some limited evidence exists to suggest re-establishment of a more posterior CR within two years of reconstruction in dentate patients.

The basic unit of centric occlusion is the *cusp/fossa* relationship, with a *supporting cusp* occluding with a *centric stop* (Fig. 7.3). The centric stop may be a fossa or a pair of marginal ridges or a single sluiceway (Fig. 7.4). Each cusp will rest in a fossa with a *tripod* relationship (Fig. 7.5), which is exceedingly difficult to reproduce in restorations. Loss of the tripod

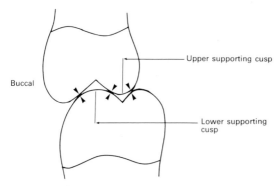

Buccal

Upper supporting cusp

Lower supporting cusp

**Fig. 7.3** Cusp/fossa relationship in bucco-lingual section. Stability is provided by the accurate meeting of the inclined planes.

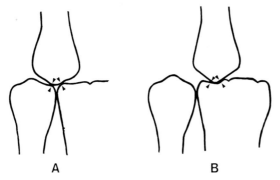

A                    B

**Fig. 7.4** Cusp/fossa relationships in mesio-distal section. The upper supporting cusp may occlude with two marginal ridges (A), or into a sluiceway (B).

contacts will lead to loss of *occlusal stability* and may induce tooth movement — over-eruption, tilting or rotation.

The discrepancy between CR and CO introduces apparent disharmonies which seem to be tolerated by the majority of people.

When closing on the terminal hinge axis or *retruded arc of closure*, there will usually be tooth contact before CO; this is the *retruded contact position* (RCP). This is followed by an anterior and upward *slide* from this first, or *premature contact*, into centric occlusion (Fig. 7.6). When closing naturally into CO, the prematurities are not contacted; it is learnt behaviour to avoid them. Closure occurs straight to CO on a favoured arc of closure.

Intrusion by stress, anxiety and so on, into the central nervous system may interfere with the co-ordination of this behaviour. This may lead to TMJ dysfunction (Ch 20).

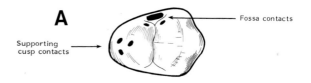

A

Fossa contacts

Supporting cusp contacts

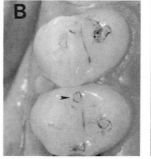 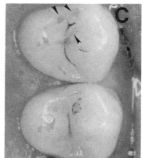

B                    C

**Fig. 7.5** Cusp/fossa relationships. **A**, Occlusal view of an upper premolar showing classic tripod contacts, one set in the sluiceway fossa and the other on the tip of the supporting cusp; **B** and **C**, Clinically this may be obscured by folding of the articulating paper in the fossae, or by natural variations in relationships. The fossa contact in **C** is almost a tripod, whilst that in **B** is a flat contact on the top of the marginal ridge.

### Mandibular guidance

The guidance of mandibular movements comes from the condyles and their relationship with the fossae (the *condylar guidance*) and the tooth to tooth contacts (*tooth guidance*). Tooth guidance is made up of *anterior/incisal guidance* and *posterior guidance*.

Because the condyles can turn *and* slide, and thus adapt to tooth positions, in practical terms, the condylar guidance is not as important as the tooth guidance.

Anterior movement from CO goes 'horizontal' at first (*long centric*) before lower incisors contact the palatal surfaces of upper incisors and the mandible has to open. It moves forward and downwards to incisal edge contact. The posterior teeth are *discluded*, but the amount of disclusion depends upon the height of the anterior guidance, the steepness of the curve of Spee, the cusp height of posterior teeth and their slopes (Fig. 7.7).

Lateral movement may be *canine guided/protected* or in *group function*. In canine guidance, the lateral movement is guided only by upper canine to lower canine contact, coupled with the condylar guidance from the non-working side condyle (Fig. 7.8).

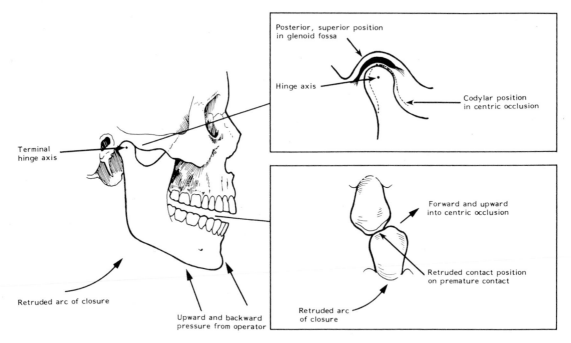

Fig. 7.6 The retruded arc of closure and a precentric premature contact on two premolars. Following this contact, the mandible slides upwards and forwards into centric occlusion.

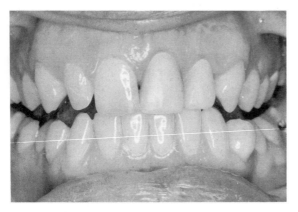

Fig. 7.7 Anterior guidance. In sliding forwards with the upper and lower incisors together, the mandible also moves downwards, discluding the posterior teeth. This patient has a high anterior guidance.

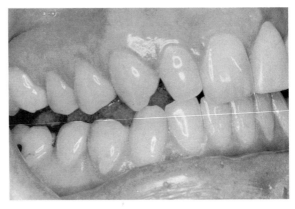

Fig. 7.8 Canine guidance. The movement of the mandible to the right and downwards is dictated by the contact of the upper and lower canines and the slope of the condylar guidance on the left, non-working side.

In group function, on the other hand, multiple contacts of the cheek teeth occur (Fig. 7.9). The popularity of group function as a restorative scheme arose from studies of primitive peoples who ate an abrasive diet, thus losing cusp tips and bringing several teeth into contact in lateral movement. This is therefore argued as the 'correct' scheme for man. However, in western races, canine guidance predominates in people under 40 years of age, whilst group function occurs after this age due to tooth wear. Therefore, to favour one scheme to the exclusion of the other would seem to be illogical. As

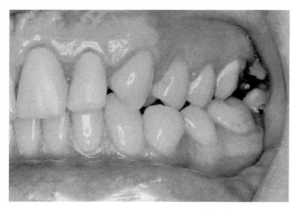

**Fig. 7.9** Group function. There are multiple contacts between the upper and lower teeth when the patient moves to the left.

will be described later, it is better to conform to the scheme already present, unless there are positive contraindications.

The condylar movement during lateral excursions, first reported by Bennett, exhibits *side-shift*. A smooth movement of the *non-working* condyle towards the *working side* is the *progressive* side-shift. There may be also a bodily movement of the mandible as soon as the lateral movement commences — the *immediate side-shift*.

Finally, just to confuse things, the teeth do not usually meet during mastication and they attain CO for swallowing only. During eating, the mandible describes some form of 'tear-drop' pathway, with a favoured chewing side. The meeting of the teeth in CO during swallowing is a critical phase, given the number of times this will occur during the day and night. In addition, *para-functional* movements, which occur with tooth contact in many positions and with no food present, require exact and accurate tooth positions if occlusal disorders are not to be provoked.

## THE PHYSIOLOGY OF MASTICATION

When an individual is at rest, with maximum relaxation of the jaw muscles, the teeth are not in contact, but are separated by the so-called *freeway space* of about 2 mm. This is the physiological rest position of the mandible. There appears to be electrical activity in the jaw muscles even when at maximum rest, suggesting that the freeway space is

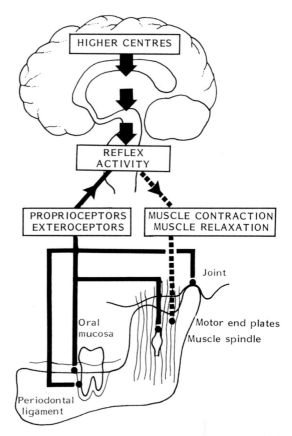

**Fig. 7.10** Neural control of mastication. Proprioceptive and exteroceptive information from the muscles and oral tissues is processed in the brain stem. Under the influence of higher centres, motor impulses are relayed to the muscle end organs.

maintained by muscle tone monitored by muscle spindles (see below), rather than by the elastic properties of the muscles and surrounding tissues.

The control of mastication is an extremely complicated activity and only the main principles can be covered here (Fig. 7.10). In so far as brain mechanisms are concerned, it appears that there are centres in the cortex, in the hypothalamus and limbic systems, and in the brain stem itself, each of which has central pathways to the trigeminal nucleus and thus controlling the muscles of mastication. In addition, the jaw movements used during speech are controlled quite separately. Disturbances in the central mechanisms controlling mandibular movements may result in clinical conditions such as bruxism (Ch. 20).

The direct control of the muscles of mastication is

via the trigeminal motor nucleus lying in the middle level of the pons. Each individual muscle is innervated by a motor neurone in a particular region of the motor nucleus.

The activity of the muscles is monitored continuously via their proprioceptive reflexes, which are largely controlled via the muscle spindles which exist in all the masticatory muscles. They are found in large numbers in the jaw elevator muscles, but much less in the depressors. The muscle spindles consist of specialized intrafusal fibres enclosed in a thin capsule and lying parallel to the main extrafusal muscle fibres or ordinary contractile fibres. Each muscle spindle contains both nuclear bag and nuclear chain fibres, the stretch in which is monitored by primary myelinated group I afferent nerves and thinner myelinated group II nerves. Stretching of the main muscle results in stretching of the muscle spindles, resulting in information being sent to the central nervous system. These spindles therefore monitor the stretch reflex of the muscles.

Information from the central nervous system and alpha efferent nerves returns to the extrafusal or main muscle fibres causing them to contract. The sensitivity of the muscle spindles is adjusted by motor innervation of the intrafusal fibres within the spindle. These consist of two types called static and dynamic fusimotor fibres, and are supplied by gamma I or gamma II nerve endings. This system means that when normal muscle tone is maintained, the spindles are detecting stretching or shortening of the muscle.

However, if the muscle contracts considerably, the spindles would no longer detect slight changes of length. At this point, the gamma motor neurones shorten the spindle so that it is again able to monitor muscle tone. Information is also sent to the central nervous system from Golgi tendon organs which are much less sensitive than muscle spindles. Information from these appears to have an inhibitory effect on the motor neurones so that the muscle spindles and Golgi tendon organs work together to maintain functional activity of the muscles.

These reflex arcs control various reflexes in the masticatory cycle. These are jaw opening reflexes, a variant of which is the horizontal jaw reflex occurring in lateral or horizontal movement.

There is also a jaw closing reflex, which 'operates' the retruded arc of closure. However, the normal path of closure is not the reflex one, but the habitual one that achieves centric occlusion efficiently.

In addition to the information from the muscle spindles and Golgi tendon organs, information is fed to the central nervous system from receptors in the joints, particularly in the capsule of the TMJ and in the peripheral parts of the articular disc. There are also receptors in the periodontium which range from non-specialized nerve endings to more complex structures. Pain is monitored via sensory nerve endings and directional sensitivity may be associated with mechano-receptors. The presence of food in the mouth is monitored by exteroceptors in the oral mucosa.

### The masticatory cycle

It seems that when food is placed in the mouth its contact with the oral mucosa initiates, through sensory nerve endings, the commencement of the masticatory cycle. The size, hardness, taste and texture of the food is appreciated and this information is processed by an 'oscillator' system in the brain stem close to the trigeminal nucleus so that rhythmic chewing movements begin. These movements are modified by reflex activity originating from nerve endings in the muscles of mastication, the periodontium, the oral mucosa and the TMJ, and are modified by the guidance planes provided by the joints, but more particularly by the teeth themselves.

When the information reaching the central nervous system suggests that the food is well comminuted and formed into a bolus, *deglutition* begins. The relevant part of this is that the mandible goes into centric occlusion to be 'locked' in that position so that the pharyngeal constrictors and the tongue can operate from a firm base, and that an anterior seal can be provided.

In such a complex system, instability of teeth, missing teeth, teeth in malocclusion or premature contact, pain in any tissues of the mouth, disturbances in the joint itself or influence from the central nervous system, frequently result in facial pain arising from either the muscles themselves or referred to the masticatory apparatus, including the joint. Clinical dental procedures are aimed at restoring the harmony between all these components of the masticatory system.

# 8. Properties of restorative materials

*G. J. Pearson   P. H. Jacobsen*

Direct restorative materials are placed into a hostile environment, and it is against the requirement to exist in this environment that they must be judged.

Ideally, the properties of the materials replacing tooth structure should be comparable to those of enamel and dentine, but the properties of the currently available materials fall short of this ideal. Present materials act merely as obturators of the holes cut in teeth. Little attempt has been made to match them, either physically or chemically, to the hard tissues they replace, and any similarities are purely coincidental.

Various physical properties of tooth tissues are shown in Table 8.1, but what these values do not reveal is the anisotropy of the tooth as a whole. It is, in fact, a very complex composite structure, and physical values vary not only with the site of the tissue, but also with the way in which it is tested.

Tooth substance is also viscoelastic, being able to deform under load and recover subsequently. The dentine is much more elastic than the enamel, which is essentially brittle. The combination of the two make a very interesting engineering structure, but with their combined constants almost impossible to determine. Add to this the elasticity of the periodontal ligament which absorbs some occlusal loading, and the puzzle is complicated even further.

Therefore, one can only sympathize with the materials scientist who is called upon to design replacements for lost or excised tissues. However, no matter how sympathetic, the clinician must judge materials by their behaviour in the mouth.

## PHYSICAL PROPERTIES OF RESTORATIVE MATERIALS

Various physical criteria may be used to describe materials and test their ability to restore teeth. Table

**Table 8.1**  Physical properties of tooth substance compared with some restorative materials

| | Enamel | Dentine | Amalgam | Composite conventional/hybrid | Cement base | Gold type III |
|---|---|---|---|---|---|---|
| Modulus of elasticity (MPa) | $4.8–4.6 \times 10^4$ | $1.4–1.2 \times 10^4$ | $1.1–2.0 \times 10^4$ | $1.4–0.7 \times 10^4$ | $0.12–0.04 \times 10^{-3}$ | $10.5–7.5 \times 10^{-4}$ |
| Compressive strength (MPa) | 386–134 (site dependent) | 282 | 510–343 | 290–210 | 172–39 | – |
| Tensile strength diametral (MPa) | 35–30 | 30–65 | 64–48 | 55–35 | 14–4.9 | 400–450 |
| Knoop hardness | 275–440 | 50–70 | 90 | 55 | 40 | 145 |
| Thermal coefficient of expansion | $11.4 \times 10^{-6}/°C$ | $8.3–5.4 \times 10^{-6}/°C$ | 25 | $17–34 \times 10^{-6}/°C$ | – | 15 |
| Thermal Diffusivity ($cm^2\ sec^{-1}$) | $4.69 \times 10^{-3}$ | $1.85 \times 10^{-3}$ | 47 (calculated) | 2.5–6.5 | $3.5 \times 10^{-3}$ | 9000 (calculated) |

**Table 8.2**  Physical properties of restorative materials

*Mechanical properties*
   Modulus of elasticity
   Creep
   Compressive strength
   Tensile strength
   Transverse strength
   Fracture toughness
   Abrasion resistance

*Physical constants*
   Coefficient of thermal expansion
   Thermal conductivity and diffusivity
   Dimensional changes on setting

*Degradation*
   Sorption and solubility
   Corrosion
   Colour stability

*Handling characteristics*
   Mixing time
   Working time
   Setting time
   Surface finishing

8.2 lists some physical properties which are often quoted to justify clinical usage.

Historically, the basis for testing was to select a group of clinically successful materials and characterize it by laboratory tests. Any new material could then be judged against the values for the materials already in use for that particular application. Unfortunately, this approach is very restrictive of new developments, and the application and significance of some standard tests is open to question.

## Mechanical properties

Mechanical properties give an indication of material quality, but the testing method may not mimic the forces applied clinically, which vary in nature, magnitude and rate of application. Whilst considerable efforts have been made to develop clinically realistic tests, these are inevitably complicated and costly.

Mechanical properties tests also give an indication of possible handling problems, in that specimen preparation is often as crucial as the method of test. If a material causes problems, inconsistent specimens and a large scatter of results will be seen. This point is illustrated by the problems of adhesion testing where clinical inconsistencies are also reflected in a very wide scatter of results in the laboratory.

*Modulus of elasticity (Young's modulus)*

This is a fundamental property which characterizes the *rigidity* of a solid in tension or compression, when it is deformed elastically. Stiff materials, such as ceramics and metals, have high elastic moduli and materials like impression rubbers have low moduli, with the polymethyl methacrylates forming an intermediate group. The modulus reflects the amount of *deformation* or *strain* a material can undergo when a certain load or stress is applied.

When stress is plotted against strain, a characteristic curve is produced (Fig. 8.1). The slope of the linear portion where stress is proportional to strain, is the modulus.

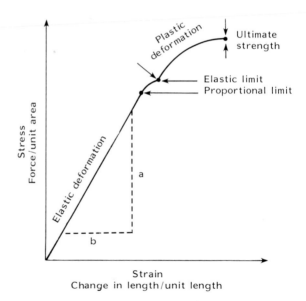

**Fig. 8.1**  Stress/strain curve. The ratio of a/b is the modulus of elasticity.

The *proportional limit* shows where the plot ceases to be linear and the *elastic limit* indicates the onset of *plastic* deformation, where the removal of the load is followed by incomplete *recovery* to the original dimensions (Fig. 8.2). Before the elastic limit, removal of the load would be followed by full recovery. If the recovery took time to occur (Fig. 8.3), the material would be *viscoelastic* and this is a characteristic of the majority of restorative materials.

Full recovery is an important property of impression rubbers after they have been removed from tooth undercuts, so that these areas are reproduced

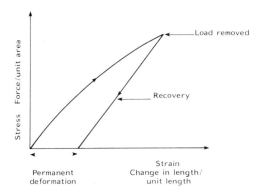

**Fig. 8.2** Stress/strain curve showing loading of a specimen past its elastic limit, resulting in a permanent deformation after the load has been removed.

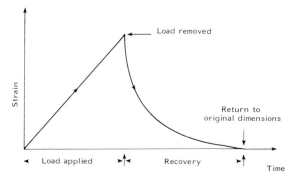

**Fig. 8.3** Strain plotted against time for a viscoelastic material. After the load has been removed, some time is necessary for full recovery to take place.

accurately. However, because of their viscoelasticity, recovery is not instantaneous, and they should not be cast for at least an hour to allow recovery to take place first. If, though, the undercuts were severe, the material would be taken beyond its elastic limit and it would not be accurate; it would have a permanent set.

On the other hand, if *ductility* is required of a metal for swaging, then the permanent deformation beyond the elastic limit, but before the *yield point*, is an essential property.

A complication of viscoelastic behaviour is that the rate at which loading takes place influences the strain, and results for modulus vary according to test conditions.

Brittle materials, such as ceramics, do not have an elastic limit, and exhibit rapid *brittle failure* when the stresses exceed the proportional limit. Viscoelastic

materials subjected to low loads which are intermittent, may eventually *fatigue*, i.e. show reduced recovery and then deteriorate by *ductile failure*.

As a concept it is important to decide which type of failure mode will occur in a given circumstance, and it is then possible to design a material for the application. As both types of failure may be seen intra-orally, depending on the material in use, design decisions are difficult, if not impossible.

Progressive permanent deformation under load is termed *creep*, and is a particular failing of dental amalgam. The loading by the occlusion causes the restoration to deform, and the margins, being thin, are the first areas to fatigue during the repeated loading. Corrosion of the metal hastens the fatigue cracking. The more successful amalgams have low creep values and lower corrosion rates. Interestingly though, the very lowest creep values do not seem advantageous, possibly because this is accompanied by brittle behaviour, with the material being too rigid to absorb stress.

Creep is measured by applying a *static* load for a given time and measuring the change in length of the specimen. However, intermittent loading is more realistic and *dynamic creep* is the manifestation of this.

### Compressive strength

This is determined by applying a steadily increasing compressive stress to a cylindrical specimen until the specimen fractures (Fig. 8.4). It might represent the loading of a restoration by the occlusion, but takes no account of the support provided by the cavity walls or absorption of stress by the periodontal ligament. Further, the incidence of compressive loading depends upon the site of the restoration, with Class III and V types receiving none.

The test gives some indication of the quality of a material but is not a definitive guide, since there is little point in having values above that of enamel, and this could be deleterious to opposing teeth.

The rate of loading of the specimen can significantly affect the results; strain rates during test of 1 mm/min are common, but apparently higher strengths can be recorded if higher rates are used. Attempts have been made to relate strain rates to those encountered during chewing, and 180 mm/min has been suggested.

## Sorption and solubility

Ideally these properties should have values of zero but the sorption of fluid by resins depends on their degree of crosslinking. Polymethyl methacrylate absorbs about 2% by weight of water and, in the long term, this decreases its strength. Other resin-based materials, such as composites, exhibit less uptake, but the amount still has a significant effect on the properties of strength and modulus of elasticity.

Similarly, there is a loss of material from most polymers with time, as the lower molecular weight compounds slowly dissolve out. The solubility decreases as the molecular weight of the resin increases and as more efficient conversion occurs during polymerization.

These properties are usually measured over a period of seven days for standard tests, but in the mouth the process continues for a considerable time until equilibrium is reached. This is frequently not for many months.

Loss of material, which tends to include plasticizers, inevitably effects the mechanical properties adversely.

Whilst water is the recognized test medium, other solvents found intra-orally, such as ethanol, and acetic and lactic acids, are likely to have deleterious effects.

The solubility values for luting cements are important as an indicator of these materials' durability. Polycarboxylates and glass ionomers, when fully matured, have the lowest values.

## Corrosion

This affects both metals and glasses, but by different mechanisms.

### Amalgam

There may be some advantage in some corrosion of amalgam since the products are bacteriocidal and also block the cavity wall/material interspace. However, the corrosion occurs in the weakest phase of the set amalgam and causes the whole structure to weaken and particularly leads to 'ditching' of the margins.

The main product of the setting reaction of conventional alloys is a cored structure of unchanged alloy powder surrounded by the silver–mercury ($\gamma_1$)

and the tin–mercury ($\gamma_2$) phases. The removal or the reduction of the latter phase has been the prime objective, since it is by far the weakest of the phases. The presence of saliva and plaque sets up corrosion cells which results in the slow breakdown of the $\gamma_2$ phase with the formation of sulphides and chlorides, and also the liberation of mercury which continues to react with the unchanged alloy.

The high copper amalgams show a marked reduction or even elimination of the $\gamma_2$ phase. The copper has a greater affinity for the tin than mercury, and copper–tin complexes are formed preferentially. These are themselves not entirely resistant to corrosion, but the rate of corrosion is considerably reduced. The end products take some time to form and the elimination of the $\gamma_2$ phase is very dependent on mercury concentration during mixing.

Corrosion and creep are all increased by the presence of excess mercury and the mixing and handling of the materials must be carefully controlled.

Certain high copper materials perform better than others and there is an overlap in performance with the poorer high coppers and the best conventional materials.

### Glasses

The ceramics employed in both composite materials as reinforcing fillers, and dental porcelains are corroded by saliva.

In the composites, water is absorbed by the resin and comes into contact with the filler. Metallic ions pass from the glass and the accumulation of corrosion products causes stress cracking in the resin. Long term immersion studies have shown dramatic decreases in strength of conventional composites. Glasses containing barium salts to confer radio-opacity are more vulnerable than alumino–silicate combinations.

However, the microfine materials are more resistant to corrosion because the filler particles are surrounded by heat cured resin which exhibits less water uptake. The clinical durability of the microfine materials is greater than would be expected from simple mechanical properties tests and this illustrates another problem in predicting clinical performance.

## Colour stability and staining

This principally applies to the resin-based materials. Loss of tooth matching colour may be due to setting reaction byproducts, degrading of the base resin or the accumulation of extrinsic stains on a degraded surface.

Amines are used as initiators in both chemically cured and light cured materials and they remain after the reaction as potential discolourants. If the amine concentration is too high, perhaps in order to accelerate setting, then colour instability will result in the long term. Accelerated ageing tests will reveal this.

The principal base resin of many composites is bis-phenol A-glycidal methacrylate (bis-GMA) and this yellows gradually when exposed to ultraviolet light. UV absorbers are added to counteract this, but they are not wholly satisfactory. The resin also changes colour due to sorption.

However, the most critical aspect of the composites is their tendency to accumulate stain on the surface. This is partly due to the degradation of the silane coupling agent which bonds the filler to the resin and partly to the abrasion of surface resin leaving a rough surface (Fig. 8.6). Porosity, which results from air inclusions during mixing and placement, also collects stain.

## Microleakage

The interface between restoration and cavity wall is an area of weakness which is under the influence of the properties discussed above. In the absence of an adhesive, mechanical interlocking between tooth and restoration is all that maintains a seal. As shrinkage and subsequent temperature changes occur, the links are broken, and fluid and bacteria pass in. The space becomes an area of transit for all types of compounds which cause staining and pulpal sensitivity. Bacteria

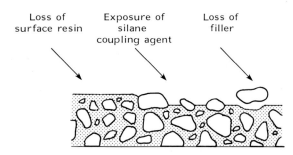

Fig. 8.6 Surface loss from a composite resin.

are the least welcome as they are able to colonize the dentine surface and are implicated in the pulpal reactions to restorative materials (Fig. 8.7).

Various techniques and materials have been developed to overcome the problem, the most successful being the cavity varnishes used with amalgam. Even these were soluble and the success of the restoration depended upon corrosion product blocking the space. The development of dentine adhesives offers the best hope for the elimination of the problem (p. 66).

Ion exchange across the interface is of considerable interest. For example, fluoride migrates from the glass ionomer cements and inhibits caries initiation at the restoration margins. The fluoride is incorporated in the glass as a flux to aid manufacture and intra-orally it slowly diffuses into the surrounding matrix from which it passes into the tooth tissue (Fig. 8.8).

## HANDLING CHARACTERISTICS

Materials must be formulated so that they can be manipulated easily. Any material that is difficult to use or is oversensitive to handling techniques is likely to be a failure, no matter how good its final properties.

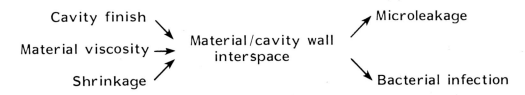

Fig. 8.7 The factors that create a material/cavity wall interspace and the consequences.

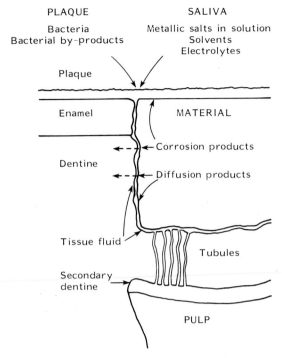

**Fig. 8.8** Microleakage. Tissue fluid together with corrosion and/or diffusion products from the material pass out and bacteria, toxins and various salts in solution pass in.

## Mixing

The most efficient way of ensuring the correct proportions of components and a satisfactory mix is to use encapsulated materials. With amalgam, encapsulation has the added advantage of improving mercury hygiene.

The cements, particularly glass ionomers, are the most sensitive to errors in proportioning and mixing. Care must be taken to follow the manufacturer's instructions exactly.

Mixing also incorporates air into the material which may lead to surface problems. Single component materials, particularly those that are vacuum packed, such as the light cured composites, help reduce the problem.

## Working time

Adequate time must be available to mix and form the restoration before the setting reaction increases the viscosity of the material to a level at which it is not workable. The chemically cured composites are the most dramatic example of this problem. They tend to be overcatalysed to please the clinician with a short setting time. Unfortunately, this severely restricts the working time leading to poor cavity wall adaptation and surface clefts if placement is not rapid.

This problem has been improved by the 'command setting' materials. These use external energy, currently light of the wavelength 410–490 nm, to excite an initiator in the material. However, the operating light also emits light of the critical wavelength, so unless it is fitted with an appropriate filter, the working time can be quite restricted.

Rapid setting amalgams, mainly spherical particle or microcut types, also have a restricted working time. If this is exceeded, increments may not amalgamate with each other, leading to 'layering' within the restoration.

## Setting time

A rapid set seems to be clinically desirable to reduce chairside time. However, this brings with it the loss of working time discussed above, and also in polymeric materials, the chain growth is restricted, leading to inferior physical properties. A long setting time can be equally deleterious, since great patience is required from the clinician. The early glass ionomer cements were very slow setting, due to the low reactivity of the glass, and early contamination with saliva leads to rapid breakdown of the restoration.

## Surface finishing

The final restoration should have very low surface energy so that it does not collect plaque and other intra-oral deposits. Often, the 'as set' material will require a finishing stage to impart a smooth surface. This must be as simple as possible and ideally done at the placement stage. However, very few materials have reached their optimum properties at this time and finishing must be delayed until maturation has occurred.

## ADHESION

A variety of attempts have been made to achieve chemical attachment of the restoration to both the enamel and dentine. Four distinct groups of adhesives have evolved, these are:

- Polycarboxylates
- Halogenated phosphate esters of bis-GMA
- Ferric mordanting systems
- Collagen grafting materials, e.g. gluteraldehyde/HEMA

The oldest adhesive system is that using polyacrylic acid as found in the polycarboxylate and glass ionomer cements. Two methods of adhesion appear to work. The first is a simple chelation reaction in which the calcium in the enamel and dentine reacts with the polyacrylate ion to form calcium polyacrylate. This requires that the surface is clean and free of pellicle. Various cleaners, or *conditioners*, have been used, starting with citric acid. This, though, produced pulpal irritation and in the last three years the use of tannic and polyacrylic acid has become more accepted. It is now thought, however, that the bond strengths to *freshly cut* dentine are no different from those found with treated dentine.

There is some chemical reaction between the organic phase of the dentine and the polyacrylate ion. This mechanism of attachment has as yet not been clearly defined but it is reported that the bond to *decalcified* dentine is very difficult to break. Though the bond strength of glass ionomer cement to dentine is not high in comparison with other adhesives, the bond appears to be the most durable and reliable of the currently available materials. It is certainly the simplest to use.

### Halogenated phosphate esters of bis-GMA

These materials are the most commonly available of the remaining adhesives and are all related chemically to the monomer used in composite resins. Bond strengths in the range 1–5 MPa have been quoted. The results are somewhat variable and depend on the type of dentine used to conduct the test and the method of test itself.

The mechanism of adhesion appears to be a linkage to the calcium in the dentine and in the smear layer produced during cavity preparation (Ch. 5). This has been confirmed by the reduction in bond strength when the smear layer is removed.

### Ferric mordanting system

This complex system has been designed to increase the metallic salts in the tooth and create a bond to this *hypermineralized* surface. This usually involves a number of stages which can be difficult to perform accurately under clinical conditions. Greater bond strengths are obtained with this material compared with the two preceding materials but currently only one commercial product has been produced and success has been variable.

### Collagen grafting systems

In these systems the dentine is reacted with materials such as acid chlorides and aldehydes and the resulting complex is reacted further with materials, such as hydroxyethylmethacrylate. The requirement of this particular system is that the smear layer and debris be cleaned away from the surface of the dentine. This is the opposite to the previously described system.

The bond strengths quoted for these materials are the highest that have been obtained but they are reduced by temperature changes.

Comparison of bis-GMA systems with glass ionomer cements suggests that the latter have better durability than the others although the bond strengths are lower. There is considerable evidence that the resin-based materials are susceptible to thermocycling and exposure to moisture. This suggests that large bond strengths are not as critical as good reliability. Also adhesion to both the organic and inorganic phases of the dentine is desirable. Adhesion to the smear layer is unpredictable.

### Methods of adhesion testing

*Bond strength*

The demonstration of effective bonding and its absolute measurement is desirable to support the efficacy of a particular system. Mechanical bond strength measurement is unfortunately fraught with potential systematic and random errors.

Forces designed to rupture the bond can be applied in several ways. The most common are tensile and shear forces (Fig. 8.9), and many individually designed test apparatuses have been proposed to apply these.

UNIAXIAL TENSION                    SHEAR

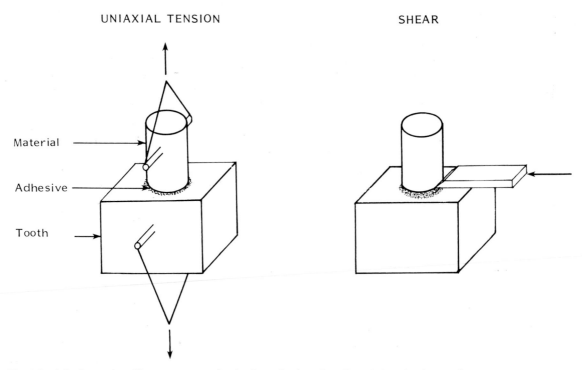

Material

Adhesive

Tooth

**Fig. 8.9** Adhesion testing. The arrangements for the determination of tensile and shear bond strengths.

Sources of error in testing may be due to the use of an incorrect substrate, surface preparation and standardization, specimen handling, and peel and shear forces created during alignment of the specimen during testing.

In view of the shortage of human teeth for testing, a number of substitutes have been used. These include animal teeth, particularly bovine, and synthetic hydroxyapatite. Both types of substitute are similar chemically to human teeth, but have structural differences. They are useful in screening potential adhesives, but finally there is no substitute for human teeth.

Variations in bond strength will also be found in parallel with compositional differences of the teeth. For example, age or position of dentine in relation to the pulp will vary the mineral content of the specimen surface.

The surface area for bonding must be carefully and accurately defined and the method must not contaminate the surface. For ease of analysis, the surface must be flat and, to avoid mechanical interlocking contributing to the bond, as plane as possible. Handling the specimen after bonding will need extreme care if the bond is not to be prematurely stressed.

A universal joint system is usually incorporated into tensile testing assemblies to align the specimen and substrate with the direction of the applied force. However, during this alignment the bond can be stressed non-axially by peel and shear forces.

*Microleakage*

The measurement of the intrusion of an agent, such as a dye, into the space between the material and the tooth is also a common test for the demonstration of adhesion. This should reflect the effects of inclusion in a cavity rather more than the simple flat surface bond strength tests.

Many intrusion agents have been used such as radio-isotopes, bacteria, electrolytes and air. However, the hydrodynamics of the dentine cannot be reproduced, and results may not correlate with clinical observations.

## BIOLOGICAL COMPATIBILITY

Biological compatibility is of paramount importance for any material that is placed permanently in living tissues. By virtue of compounds leaching from the material, local or systemic effects are possible.

Dental materials are often placed at a time when they are chemically active, after which they set and become essentially inert. A series of in vitro and in vivo tests have been devised to screen the biological properties of restorative materials.

The in vitro tests begin with a simple screening of cell cytotoxicity, after which the material will be tested in animals. The animal tests are of implantation in the tissues and simulated in-use tests in the teeth. The material is placed in standardized cavities and the pulpal response noted at various time intervals after placement. There are a number of problems with this test in terms of reproducibility and variability but, in the absence of any reliable alternative, it is the best guide to compatibility for restorative materials. The laboratory tests at the cellular level tend to eliminate materials which are acceptable in other tests. For instance, the cytotoxicity is reduced if fully set material is used instead of freshly mixed material.

The presence or absence of an intervening layer of dentine between material and pulp alters the response of pulp tissue to the material very considerably. Zinc oxide eugenol cements are the classic example of this, in that if they are applied to exposed pulp, they induce inflammation, whilst they are obtundent to the closed pulp.

## CLINICAL TESTING

Following laboratory testing, the materials are subjected to clinical trials. An initial *explanatory trial* using controlled conditions and a small number of clinicians, is followed by a *field trial* in which the material is used by many operators in general practice conditions.

The time scale for these assessments is inevitably long and costly. It might be as long as five years between invention of a material and its marketing, but there is no avoiding this. Realistic accelerated tests are difficult to devise in primates and not representative of human intra-oral conditions.

## SUMMARY

The combination of laboratory tests, animal studies and clinical trials ought to provide the clinician with considerable valuable information on the likely behaviour of a material when it is placed in the mouth.

Unfortunately this is not the case, since there are so many unquantifiable biological factors which influence clinical success. Not least of these is the skill of the clinician in handling materials. Proper attention to detail and the understanding of the quirks of each material is an essential component of the dentist's education.

# Clinical and technical procedures

# 9. Intracoronal restorations

*G. J. Pearson*

It is nearly a century since G. V. Black produced his original guidelines on cavity preparation which formed the mainstay of conservative dentistry for many years.

However, materials, cutting instruments and techniques have since evolved to a considerable degree, and this, together with a better understanding of the structure of the dental hard and soft tissues and of the carious disease process, has resulted in modifications to the principles of cavity design.

Black's original concepts arose partly as a result of the cutting instruments of his day. Removal of hard tissue with burs and pedal engines was slow and difficult, which led to lesions not being treated until they were of considerable size. By this time, caries had usually spread beneath the enamel until this had fractured away. Thus, the outline form of the cavity was almost always predetermined by the disease process rather than the need to preserve tooth tissue. The problem was compounded by the necessity for using large diameter burs in order that higher peripheral cutting speeds could be obtained to achieve greater efficiency. In addition, the original cavities were designed for gold foil, and only minor modifications were made for amalgam, which is, of course, a very different material.

Today, the advent of adhesive materials coupled with the more precise diagnosis of caries by radiography, has led to different designs. The need for retention created by the cavity shape has been reduced and the lesion is treated at a much earlier stage.

## INDICATIONS FOR TREATMENT

There is considerable evidence to support the

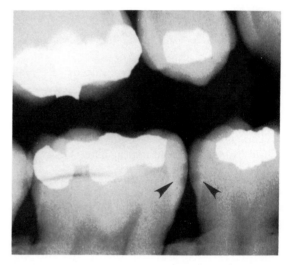

**Fig. 9.1** Bitewing radiograph showing early enamel caries (arrowed) which should receive topical fluoride application, rather than restoration.

remineralization of the early carious lesion in enamel. Only when the lesion shows positive evidence of having reached the dentine, should operative treatment be commenced. Figure 9.1 shows a radiograph of an early lesion for which the application of topical fluoride coupled with regular radiographic review would be appropriate.

Figure 9.2, on the other hand, shows clear evidence of caries in dentine, and this lesion should be excised. In relation to the diagnosis of caries, it is very important to be aided by good quality radiographs which have been taken and processed by standardized techniques.

The extent of the excision and the final shape of the cavity depend upon:

- The size of the lesion
- Its position with regard to aesthetics

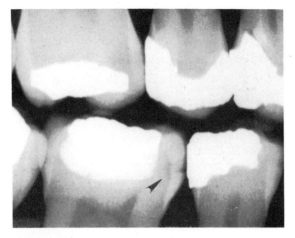

**Fig. 9.2** Bitewing radiograph showing an approximal carious lesion (arrowed) which extends into dentine. This lesion should be excised and the tooth restored.

- The need to conserve tooth substance
- The choice of restorative material
- Caries incidence and oral hygiene

The *choice of restorative material* is central to the whole cavity design process. Does it need to be tooth coloured, is it going to be in occlusal function, how large is the lesion?

Low *caries incidence* and good *oral hygiene* would indicate very conservative cavity designs with minimal extension.

## TREATMENT OF THE MINIMAL DENTINE LESION

### Occlusal caries — the preventive resin restoration

The minimal lesion in an occlusal fissure should be treated by local excision of the carious dentine, through the overlying enamel. The access should be of sufficient size to allow good vision of the affected dentine. The other fissures on the occlusal aspect should be inspected for evidence of caries, rather than just staining, and should not be removed unless carious dentine can be seen under them. Occlusal stops will be unlikely to be removed by such a preparation, and therefore glass ionomer cement (GIC) can be used because of its good adhesion to dentine, low pulp irritation and fluoride exchange (Ch. 8).

The remainder of the fissure pattern should be acid etched prior to the insertion of the GIC, and fissure sealed after insertion. The fissure sealant should be extended over the GIC to protect it from water (Fig. 9.3).

If the fissure is very steep, so that the sealant will not enter it fully, or there is suspicious staining, then *fissure widening* may be used. A fine tapered diamond is run along the fissure at the depth of the enamel–dentine junction. Any caries revealed by this can be removed locally by a small round bur, run at

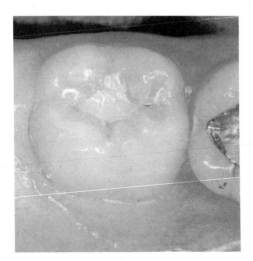

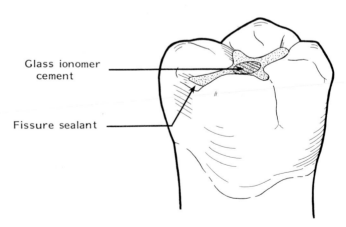

Glass ionomer cement

Fissure sealant

**Fig. 9.3** The preventive resin restoration. The deeper part of the cavity is filled with glass ionomer cement, and this, plus the fissure system, has acid etch resin applied to it.

slow speed. The whole cavity can now be restored with GIC, or acid etch retained composite resin.

## Approximal caries

There are several miniscule designs which have been suggested (Fig. 9.4). All of these rely on very precise control of fine cutting instruments, and the unique properties of glass ionomer cement. It is also essential to use magnification for accurate vision whilst cutting.

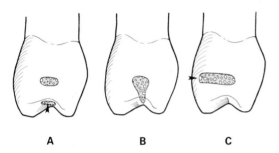

**Fig. 9.4** Microcavities. **A** shows the tunnel preparation where access (arrowed) is obtained through the occlusal surface, under the marginal ridge to the approximal caries. **B** allows direct vision of the approximal caries and **C** is the lateral approach (arrowed) from the buccal aspect.

The *tunnel* preparation (Fig. 9.4A) maintains the marginal ridge, but care must be taken not to touch the adjacent tooth as the tunnelling emerges approximally. Sight of the approximal lesion is obtained by widening the occlusal access buccolingually. GIC is suitable for small lesions; in the larger cavity it can be used for the approximal part, but it may be surfaced with composite resin occlusally.

The *lateral* approach (Fig. 9.4C) gains its access to the lesion from the embrasure on the buccal aspect using a round diamond instrument. This relies on the accurate diagnosis of the size of the lesion, since anything above very small results in a considerably larger cavity than the minimum required because of the orginal restricted access.

## MODERATE LESIONS

### Selection of restorative material

This has a direct influence on the size and shape of cavity to be cut, and in turn is influenced by the site and size of the original lesion. The material of choice in the posterior teeth is amalgam, and that where aesthetics is of prime concern is composite resin.

However, the use of composite resin in posterior teeth must be viewed with caution since it is technically more demanding than amalgam and may not maintain occlusal contacts as well.

The *cervical lesion* may be restored with composite resin or GIC if it is bounded by enamel, and by GIC if it is sited in dentine. In this region, the composite currently provides the best aesthetics and bonds well to acid etched enamel, whilst the GIC has durable bonding to dentine, but has the important advantages of fluoride exchange and better stain resistance. Where cervical root caries has appeared in areas of gingival recession, or in sensitive abrasion cavities, GIC is the material of choice.

Because the adhesion of both composite resin and GIC is variable, it is unwise to rely on it totally for retention, and mechanical undercuts must be provided. However, as was discussed in Chapter 8, marginal leakage is considerably reduced.

Gold inlays are very much out of favour. The skills required, coupled with the weakness of the cement lute, make them inferior in the majority of operator's hands to the average amalgam restoration. This is not to say that the placement of amalgam does not require a high level of skill, it does, but the technique is more forgiving.

## Instrumentation

Limits on the extent of cavity preparation are imposed by the bur dimensions, the precision and state of the handpiece bearing and the visual acuity of the operator.

### Burs

Burs used may be divided into those which *abrade* away the surface and those which *cut* the surface. The first category includes the diamond instruments which have a fine grit of diamond embedded in the matrix of the bur. Their method of production limits their effective diameter to not less than 0.8 mm, and the wear on a bur of such a size is very rapid. These abrade away the surface of the dentine producing a surface of uniform roughness (Fig. 9.5).

Tungsten carbide burs have blades with cutting

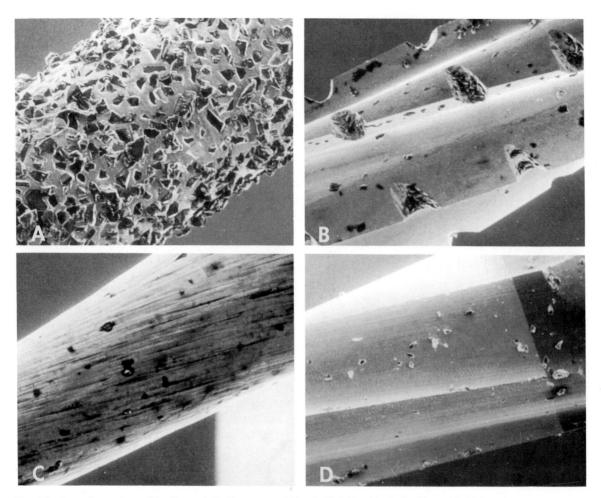

**Fig. 9.5**  Burs: the surfaces of **A**, diamond; **B**, Tungsten carbide; **C**, Finishing blank; **D**, The welded joint of a tungsten carbide bur, which is an area of weakness.

edges which may be serrated to increase the cutting rate. Here again there is a limit to how narrow these burs can be before the risk of fracture of the metal becomes unacceptable, and they are restricted to diameters greater than 0.8 mm. At any thickness, though, they are very prone to fracture if any lateral stress is placed on them. This fracture will be either at the shank or within the structure of the bur itself, depending on the design (Fig. 9.5).

This limitation plus the eccentricity of the handpiece means that the minimum possible width of cavity which can be obtained realistically is about one millimetre.

Burs with a sharp terminal profile, such as the inverted cone or flat fissure, introduce stress con-

centrations in the line angles of a cavity, and round profile burs, such as the dome fissure, are preferred.

### Conservative class II cavity

Apart from actually removing the caries, the over-riding considerations are to conserve as much tooth substance as possible and to provide mechanical stability for the restoration.

### Occlusal section

The *occlusal key* is cut to one-quarter to one-fifth the intercuspal distance (Fig. 9.6), which reduces to a

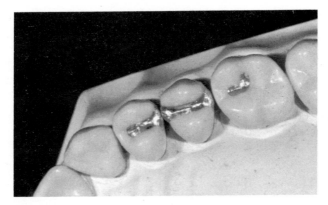

**Fig. 9.6**  Conservative cavities for amalgam.

minimum the risk of weakening the remaining tooth structure.

Any further reduction in cavity width here is determined by the restorative material which has been chosen. Adequate space must be provided for the entry of the amalgam condenser, though less is required for composite resins, since they flow under pressure.

The cavity design should avoid cutting enamel centric stops since none of the direct materials is capable of maintaining occlusal stability over long periods. In particular, evidence to date suggests that the successful use of composites and glass ionomers in the posterior region requires that they are placed in non-stress bearing areas. Also, freehand carving of accurate occlusal morphology is unreliable (Ch. 7).

The extent of the caries may prevent such minimal outlines, but as a general rule and where possible, adoption of this principal would extend the life expectancy of any restoration.

The cavity should extend just below the enamel–dentine junction occlusally, so that this may be inspected for caries and the restoration can be based on dentine, which has more resilience. Localized areas of caries should be removed either with excavators or slow running large round burs. The irregularities in the floor of the cavity can be filled later with some form of structural base.

The extension of the cavity into the fissures and embrasures should be determined by the patient's predisposition to caries, and with a large number of carious lesions in fissures, fissure extension would be advisable. The tooth morphology would also affect the decision. Deep convoluted fissures will pre-dispose towards recurrence of caries and could be excised.

*Approximal section*

One of the main problems associated with the approximal box preparation is a failure to determine the site of the carious lesion in all three planes prior to the commencement of the preparation. The tendency is to cut standard shaped cavities without locating the lesion properly, which results in extension either too far lingually or buccally. Slightly rotated teeth are a particular problem. The initial penetration of the marginal ridge should be made directly towards the lesion, and not simply to remove the entire proximal surface in one go.

The margins of the preparation should just clear the contact with the adjacent tooth, buccally, lingually and cervically, meaning that the outline follows the embrasure shape, though with straight edges. The box profile is therefore naturally undercut (Fig. 9.7).

Clearing the contact means that the restoration margins are accessible for finishing and for oral hygiene. It also allows a matrix to be placed (p. 81).

*Stability*

In spite of the advances in adhesives, it is unwise to rely on any of the current types to provide stability for class II restorations. Conventional retention is still required to prevent displacement, by having the base of the cavity fractionally wider than the outline which

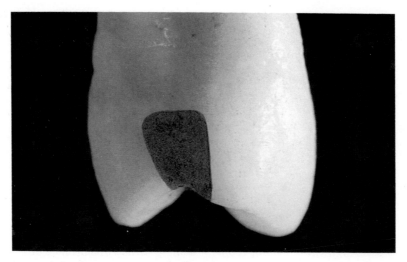

**Fig. 9.7** Approximal box outline for a conservative cavity.

provides a mechanical key, and having a flat floor for stability.

The approximal box requires resistance to prevent displacement towards the adjacent tooth, and this should be provided by the occlusal portion of the cavity.

When using composite resins, microleakage is reduced by the bond to acid etched enamel. To achieve this bond, prisms must be etched in their long axis and bevelled margins are necessary to expose prism ends in certain areas. The proximal box margins should be bevelled, but not the occlusal section. Here the enamel is cut transversely by the normal preparation because of its slope towards the fissure.

### Anterior restorations

Here all that is required is excision of the lesion with the minimum removal of tooth substance. The old kidney shaped class V cavity is quite unnecessary.

It is desirable to adopt a palatal approach for the approximal lesion wherever possible for aesthetic reasons, and to angle the bur into the lesion under the marginal ridge to maintain enamel in the occlusion (Fig. 9.8). The labial extension should be just through the contact, and whilst this may result in a very thin layer of enamel and dentine or enamel alone, the modern aesthetic materials offer the advantage of supporting this layer through bonding; this produces

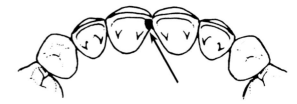

**Fig. 9.8** Direction of access to a mesial lesion on an incisor. The marginal ridge is preserved by this line of approach.

a better aesthetic result. The necessity for the palatal extensions or dovetails frequently included in the older class III cavities has been obviated by the advent of the acid etch technique and the newer dentine adhesives. As with the class II, though, it is still preferable to include some mechanical retention as well. This would take the form of gingival and incisal pits and grooves, providing these do not weaken the remaining tooth.

The choice of restorative material is between GIC and composite resin, with the GIC having an advantage in individuals with high caries rates.

Where teeth are to be restored with composite resin, a bevel applied to all enamel margins will improve the etching characteristics, but will result in a thin wedge of composite resin at the periphery of the restoration. If the bond fails, chipping and staining will occur and so it might be better to avoid bevelling, provide mechanical retention and use the

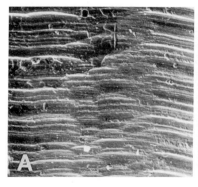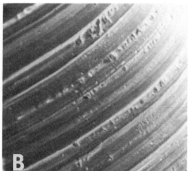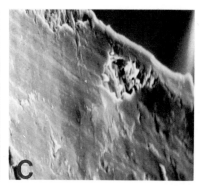

**Fig. 9.9**   The surfaces created by various finishing burs: **A**, Diamond; **B**, Tungsten carbide; **C**, White stone, showing a smear layer. (Field width 250 μm.)

acid etch technique to improve marginal adaptation only.

### Cavity finishing

Differing opinions exist as to whether cavity walls should be left as they are cut or smoothed with some form of blank (Fig. 9.5) or multi-bladed finishing bur. The surface produced by different burs is striking (Fig. 9.9), but did not seem to be critical for clinical results until the arrival of adhesives.

The quality of the adhesive bond is dependent to a large extent on the morphology of the substrate to which it is applied; this will vary according to the instruments used. The rougher the surface, the more difficult will be the wetting of this by the adhesive. The result will be air pockets under the restoration which will be a route for microleakage, in spite of the adhesive. So the smoother the surface, the more efficient will be the adhesive process.

The cutting of both enamel and dentine produces a layer of amorphous material which is smeared over the surface of the enamel and dentine (the *smear layer*) which is rich in calcium. The amount of smear created depends on the type of bur used. The ranking order from most to least is white stone, blank, diamond and tungsten carbide burs. The tenacity of the smear layer has never been determined, but it appears to be relatively weak. Its presence confers two advantages:

- Sealing of the dentinal tubules
- Provision of a calcium rich layer

The smear layer blocks the cut ends of the dentinal tubules, and therefore may be a factor in protecting the pulp from microleakage.

The increase in the surface calcium will be of use with many of the adhesive systems which bond to the inorganic component of the tooth. However, it is a problem with materials which bond to organic constituents such as collagen. One of the requirements for these materials is the removal of the smear layer to expose the organic component, but opening of the dentinal tubules might result in damage to the underlying odontoblastic processes. The *conditioners* used for adhesive techniques have been discussed in Chapter 8.

A number of cavity cleansers have been proposed for use with amalgam. Some of these have proved harmful, such as the dehydrating alcohol varieties. The blander ones are designed to remove bacteria, which have been implicated in pulpal reactions under restorations. This may be desirable, but they also remove the smear layer which is better left alone. The best and most biologically acceptable cleanser for use prior to placing amalgam seems to be the air and water from the triple syringe.

### PULP PROTECTION — LININGS

On completion of the cavity a decision should be made regarding the need for further pulpal protection. In the majority of minimal cavities, the protection afforded by the dentine from both chemical and mechanical irritation is adequate, but once the cavity extends beyond minimal size, additional pulpal protection is required.

Lining materials may be divided into three groups:

- Bases
- Liners
- Varnishes

## Bases

The primary purpose of these materials is to protect the pulpal tissue from mechanical and chemical irritation. Their properties also allow their use as a dentine replacement. They are usually used in thick section to act as thermal insulators.

For clinical use, it is important that they reach a substantial strength quickly, otherwise the restoration placement, particularly the condensation of amalgam, will be unsatisfactory.

### Zinc phosphate cement

This material is still used routinely by some operators as a base since it is easy to manipulate. The main constituents are buffered phosphoric acid and a mixture of zinc oxide and magnesium oxide, and it sets by the formation of a hydrated zinc phosphate.

Biologically, there are reservations about the cement since a considerable amount of free acid remains for some time after mixing. This may be responsible for pulpal irritation and pulpal necrosis, but bacterial ingress might be more important. Its other main drawback is its susceptibility to fluid contamination, especially during the early stages of setting.

The cement is stronger than any of the other bases in compression and therefore provides stability in thick section when the restoration is placed.

### Zinc polycarboxylate cement

More recent developments of bases have centred on the polycarboxylate cements. Again the powder consists of a mixture of zinc oxide and magnesium oxide, with polyacrylic acid and co-polymers as the original liquid. This has now been superseded by vacuum dried polyacrylic acid incorporated in the powder, which is simply mixed with water. The resulting material, which has a zinc polyacrylate matrix, has similar properties to those of phosphate cement, but its main advantage is that it possesses adhesive properties to tooth structure. Pulpal irritation is reported to be significantly below that of phosphate cement, which may be due to the high molecular weight of the polyacrylic acid. The material is therefore rather better than phosphate cement, but it has more difficult handling characteristics.

### Zinc oxide eugenol (ZOE) cements

These are derived from the original simple ZOE cement which was used as a sedative dressing. In its crudest form the material was not strong enough to be used as a base or as a long term temporary dressing. It did, however, have an obtundent effect on pulp symptoms as long as dentine remained over the pulp. On exposed soft tissue, the material is an irritant.

The basic ZOE cements have been modified by the addition of a variety of materials. Zinc stearate and zinc acetate were first included as a means of increasing the strength and shortening the setting time, and either polystyrene or ethoxybenzoic acid have been added to reinforce the materials further.

Whilst still the weakest of the bases, mixed correctly it provides good service. However, incorrect proportioning is common, which means that the material is used below its optimum properties.

The importance of having a strong base has been demonstrated by work which shows that there is a displacement of the restoration under load and that the displacement is directly related to the type of cement used as a base.

The other disadvantage of the eugenol based materials is that they are not compatible with all restorative materials. Resin based materials are plasticized by the eugenol and their polymerization is retarded.

## Liners

These materials form a thin layer over the pulpal floor of deep cavities; the commonest forms are the calcium hydroxide cements whose therapeutic action is discussed in Chapter 10. The calcium hydroxide is combined with a resin base which may be chemically cured or light activated.

Chemically cured liners have poor mechanical properties in comparison with the bases discussed earlier, but they are valuable as chemical insulators in shallow cavities and as sublinings in deep ones. In deep cavities, they should always be covered by a structural base because of their weakness.

The development of light activated resin based liners has changed the materials considerably. Their advantage is the increase in the mechanical properties, but there is a reduction in the pH of the cement from 11 to 7 and this property influences secondary dentine deposition, which is reduced. It is possible that these materials will not be as effective as pulp capping agents.

**Cavity varnishes**

These materials are usually based on resins such as copal varnish and polystyrenes in a volatile solvent. Their main purpose is to prevent the ingress of bacteria and microleakage into the dentine tubules. They are not thermal insulators, and have high solubility.

They have been replaced in anterior restorations by the adhesives, and their long term durability with amalgam is questionable.

## MATRICES

A plethora of matrix retainers and bands is available and it is difficult to single out any one particular type as being the ideal. However, there are a number of desirable features in any system:

- The approximal contour should be reproduced accurately
- The band should be thin enough to provide an adequate contact and yet be rigid enough not to buckle or crease
- The bands must be of sufficient variety to match various tooth shapes
- The retainer should be stable and allow correct tightening of the band at the cervical margin
- For light cured materials, the bands must allow transmission of light

The difficulties of all the current systems are that none of them produce the concavo-convex outline of the natural tooth and most produce a flat surface with the contact usually at the marginal ridge rather than one-third of the way down the approximal surface.

The Siqveland type is usually the easiest to use but will produce a poorly contoured approximal surface unless it is burnished to shape. It should also be cut after packing, so that it can be removed laterally through the contact. If this is not done, there is a danger that removal will take the marginal ridge with it.

It is essential to wedge all bands, and failure to do this will result in overhangs which are difficult to remove in amalgam but almost impossible to remove with composite resins without damaging the tooth. The choice and use of wedges is also important. The wedge must hold the band against the cervical margin of the cavity. Frequently this is not achieved and the wedge rests on the margin interfering with the contour (Figs 9.10 and 9.11).

Matrices for the anterior region are ill-developed, and improper use can ruin the restoration. The most difficult restoration is the class V, since the acute convexity of the buccal aspect together with the

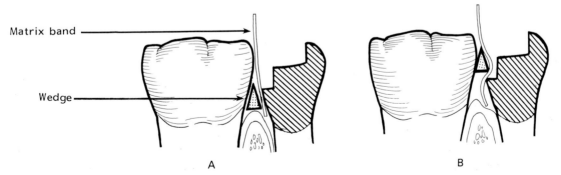

Matrix band

Wedge

A          B

**Fig. 9.10** Wedging technique. **A** shows the correct position for the wedge, and **B** shows it too high, buckling the band.

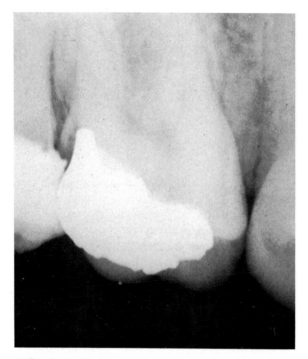

**Fig. 9.11**   Radiograph showing the result of Fig. 9.10B.

complex shape in the longitudinal plane of the teeth will frequently result in poor contour. The contoured soft metal matrices are the most satisfactory, but are unusable with light cured composites.

## RESTORATIVE MATERIALS — HANDLING

### Amalgam

The variables which can seriously alter the properties of the material and the durability of the restoration are:

- Proportioning
- Mixing
- Condensation
- Carving
- Polishing

#### Proportioning

For hand mixing it was necessary to use an excess of mercury, with mercury : alloy ratios of 8 : 5 or 7 : 5, and even after condensation, excess mercury remains, with consequent reduction in physical properties. This problem has been reduced considerably by mechanical mixing and encapsulation which, because it is more efficient, requires a ratio of about 1 : 1.

#### Mixing

The correct ratio must be mixed for the correct time. The quality of the mix will show an undermixed amalgam by its being dry and crumbly. The ideally mixed material should be a cohesive ball which can be pushed to thin film without breaking up, with the overmixed material being soupy, difficult to remove from the capsule and frequently hot to touch. Overmixing reduces the working time and increases creep values, whilst undermixing leads to an unusable mix.

#### Condensation

Undercondensation by using inadequate pressure or a large surface area condenser will result in inadequate expression of excess mercury and also lead to microporosity. Here the admixed and spherical particle alloys show some advantage, since they may be condensed with less pressure, and puddling of the alloy produces a satisfactory restoration. In fact, the use of a small condenser is contra-indicated with these alloys as the tip will push through the amalgam and leave sub-surface porosities. Mechanical condensation is also disadvantageous.

#### Carving

Correct reproduction of the occlusal contacts, together with removal of the mercury-rich excess layer, is essential. In Chapter 7, the difficulty of reproducing exact anatomical cusp/fossa relationships was described. Occlusal stability can be achieved, together with axial loading of the tooth, by carving flat centric stops to receive the opposing supporting cusps, rather than attempting tripods (Fig. 12.20). If the tripods have one or more contacts missing, the tooth will move to find stable position. This may create occlusal interferences.

The amalgam restoration should hold shimstock, and if it does then a shiny mark, or marks, will be seen on its surface; this is not necessarily a 'high spot', and an amalgam with no shiny marks will be out of occlusion. Unfortunately, the majority are taken out of occlusion for this reason and occlusal instability ensues.

## Polishing

Polishing should correct any carving errors, such as excess at the margins or occlusal problems, but not eliminate the occlusal stops already produced.

When using finishing burs or polishing pastes, it is undesirable to produce local hot spots on the surface since this will probably cause changes in the phases of the amalgam. It will also cause excess mercury to come to the surface and this will in turn weaken the material.

## Toxicity

A number of unnecessary concerns have been expressed about amalgam. While it is necessary for both the operator and dental surgery assistant to exercise care in storage and handling the material, suggestions that amalgam restorations are responsible for systemic disease cannot be substantiated scientifically or medically.

Many of the hazards in the surgery may be overcome by the use of encapsulated materials and care in the disposal of waste.

## Composite resins

These materials have made considerable advances in the last few years. The principal developments have been in filler technology with the hybrid materials, and in command setting with the light activated materials. Improved filler/resin coupling, which increases surface stability, has also been achieved.

### Light activated materials

Table 9.1 lists the advantages and disadvantages of the light activated materials. The chemically cured materials have the severe disadvantage of a very short working time which limits clinical handling. Whilst the light cured materials are affected by the operating light, the use of a yellow filter provides a considerable extension of the working time (Ch. 8).

The by-products of the amine–peroxide che-

**Table 9.1** Advantages and disadvantages of light activated materials

| Advantages | Disadvantages |
| --- | --- |
| Command setting | Depth of cure |
| Extended working time | Shadowing by tooth |
| Better colour stability | Affected by operating light |
| Improved monomers | Light source required |
| Void free | |

mical curing system lead to colour instability, and in light activated materials there is no peroxide, and the amine concentration is reduced. In addition, the manufacturer has more flexibility in the production of the material, and multi-functional monomers are common. These have enhanced physical properties.

The single component of the light activated materials can be packed under vacuum and also mixing is not required, thus eliminating air inclusions.

The disadvantages all influence clinical techniques. The restoration must be built in individually cured increments no more than about 2 mm thick. The activating light intensity falls off if it is obstructed by tooth or is some distance away from the material, as with the floor of the approximal box in a class II restoration. The depth of cure is also reduced by a darker shade.

The other variable which can seriously affect polymerization is the light source. The light output from each commercially available light varies and this can seriously affect the curing potential of the system. It may also be affected by variations in the power supply voltage which reduce the energy emitted in the critical wavelengths. A reduction in the voltage shifts the energy distribution toward the higher wavelengths. The bulb also requires changing once a year to maintain efficiency, and the continuity of fibres in the fibre optic type should also be checked. Devices are now available for testing the light output and it is worth doing this regularly.

### Posterior materials

The placement of composite resin in a class II cavity requires meticulous completion of each stage in turn, and consequently much time. The sequence of placement, which should be done under rubber dam, is:

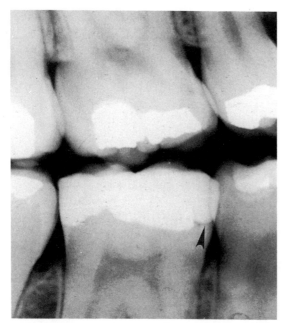

**Fig. 9.12** Bitewing radiograph of 6| restored with posterior composite. There is a failure of adaptation at the mesial cervical margin (arrowed).

1. Pre-wedge to open contact area;
2. Prepare cavity with rounded line angles and bevelled approximal box;
3. Line with non-eugenol base;
4. Acid etch enamel, apply thin layer of 'bonding agent';
5. Place transparent matrix, re-wedge;
6. Apply and cure 0.5 mm of composite at the cervical margin to avoid shrinkage and marginal failure (Fig. 9.12);
7. Build and cure remainder in 2 mm increments;
8. Complete occlusal surface.

The occlusion is difficult to restore, as free-hand carving leaves an oxygen inhibited surface which should be cut back. This may be avoided by over-filling and cutting back after curing, but this is tedious. An occlusal index can be prepared pre-operatively to mould the composite, or, rubber dam permitting, the patient can close into CO with the composite covered with a piece of cling film. This latter technique gives a quick and simple guide to the occlusal stops.

There is a higher incidence of post-operative pain following composite placement. The polymerization

shrinkage causes cuspal flexure and marginal leakage, and the light is a potent source of heat. Some materials stick to instruments and are thus pulled away from cavity floors, leading to leakage (Fig. 9.12).

## Glass ionomer cements (GIC)

These materials provide an alternative to composite resins under certain circumstances. Their solubility, translucency and general handling characteristics have been improved dramatically since the earliest materials. The advantages of GICs are their adhesion to tooth substance and their fluoride leach which have been discussed in Chapter 8.

Two distinct lines of development have been

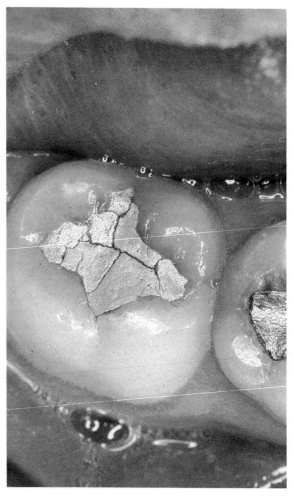

**Fig. 9.13** A glass ionomer cermet which has cracked due to water contamination.

pursued. One group have adopted the use of polyacrylic–polymaleic copolymer and encapsulation. The other approach has been to adopt the vacuum dried polyacrylic acid which is mixed with the glass and then activated by the addition of water. Adjustments have been made to give setting times of the order of 4–6 minutes. This is comparable with the majority of the chemically cured composites. The reduction in the setting time has produced a marked reduction in the solubility and sorption.

All the materials are very sensitive to water contamination in the early stages of setting, and placement should be done under rubber dam. However a certain amount of water is required, and they must not be allowed to dry out, otherwise they will crumble (Fig. 9.13).

Encapsulated materials, which are mechanically mixed, provide a much more reliable and consistent material since the method of mixing is the greatest problem with GICs at present. Poor results are usually due to incorrect proportioning and mixing, and the materials are often blamed rather than the operator's or assistant's inability to follow the instructions.

Attempts to achieve radio-opacity have been made with varying degrees of success. The majority have been associated with the addition of materials that are radio-opaque but play no part in the chemical reaction. Zinc glass is an example which imparts radio-opacity but the materials are not stable and appear to degrade. Another method is to sinter silver with the glass during its production to form a cermet.

The cariostatic properties are advantageous. Fluoride ions in the glass slowly leach out into the filling matrix and thence to the surrounding tissue. There is some suggestion that there is a reverse flow and it is now inferred from this that the GICs may act as reservoirs for various ions. This is of potential significance since it has been demonstrated that there is caries inhibition around these restorations.

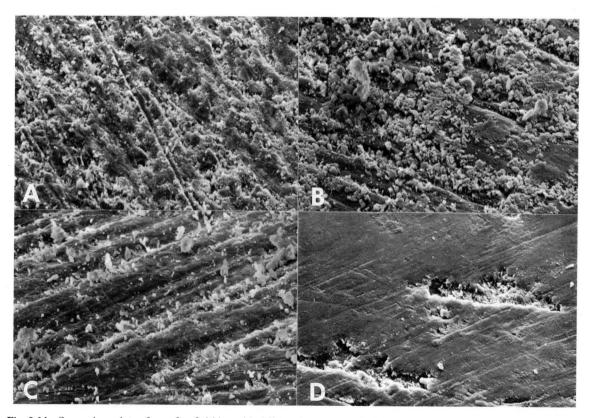

**Fig. 9.14** Composite resin surfaces after finishing with different instruments: **A**, White stone; **B**, Coarse aluminium oxide disc; **C**, Medium aluminium oxide disc; **D**, Fine aluminium oxide disc.

*Laminate (sandwich) technique*

This creates a restorative combination of GIC and composite resin which is supposed to overcome some of the inherent disadvantages of each material. The GIC brings dimensional stability, adhesion and cariostatic properties, and the composite resin brings greater strength.

The laminated restoration has GIC as its base, replacing lost dentine, with composite as its enamel surface. The mechanical bond between the two materials is created by an intermediate resin.

The system has been tried on the cervical floor of class II restorations to eliminate leakage there, and for abrasion cavities. Because the handling properties of both materials are critical, success has been variable and the technique is inevitably time consuming. The requirement is really for a stronger GIC.

## Finishing of composite resins and GIC

These materials cannot be polished, and any instrumentation of the surface after setting will produce roughness. The best surface is formed against a matrix strip, but if trimming is required, first it should be delayed for at least 12 hours so that the material is harder, and secondly the abrasive used should be appropriate.

White alpine stones or diamonds produce the roughest surfaces, whilst fine aluminium oxide impregnated discs produce the smoothest (Fig. 9.14).

## INTRACORONAL RESTORATIONS— SUMMARY

Techniques for small restorations have changed dramatically in the last few years. Advances in the diagnosis of caries, materials and cavity design have eclipsed Black's original concepts. Understanding the pathology of caries, the anatomy of the tooth and the properties of restorative materials is essential for the design of modern cavities.

Tooth tissue should be regarded as a precious resource, only to be removed if essential. Small cavities cause less trauma and do less harm to the occlusion. The restorative materials must be used within their limitations.

# 10. Management of the deep cavity

*G. J. Pearson*

In distinction from the treatment of the small to moderate carious lesion, the deep cavity requires not only a decision on the restorative technique to be used, but also, and most importantly, an assessment of the state of the pulp.

Clinical assessment of pulp conditions can be unreliable, and for this reason it is far preferable to institute regular and routine six monthly examinations to avoid, amongst other things, the problems of managing deep caries. This is particularly important in the young patient, where there is less mineralization of the dentine, and the response of the pulp to carious attack cannot keep pace with the advancing lesion. In the older patient the rate of spread is slower, and the pulpal response of laying down secondary dentine and increasing the mineral content of the dentine, is able to provide some chance of pulp defence (Ch. 6).

## PULP ASSESSMENT

There is very little information to guide the clinician in assessing the pulp, since there is no opportunity to biopsy the diseased tissue. Therefore, the fullest use needs to be made of:

* Symptoms
* Clinical appearance
* Vitality tests
* Radiographic appearance

The correlation of symptoms with pulpal pathology is poor. However, the following sequence may act as a guide:

1. Transient low grade pain on eating sweet foods — early lesion in dentine, pulp normal;
2. Transient mild pain on hot and cold foods —

deeper lesion in dentine, pulp normal;
3. More severe pain lasting after the stimulus has gone — pulp pathology.

Provided the symptoms are transient, it is fairly certain that the pulp tissue is not involved in the pathology, and the response can be regarded as essentially physiological. It is only if the pain continues after the stimulus is removed that there is a strong possibility that the pulp has started to respond at a cellular level. The more severe the pain, the less chance there is of pulp recovery after removal of the caries (Ch. 6).

Of course, this nicely ordered picture may not be seen, since the chronic nature of the lesion may not give rise to symptoms at all. Alternatively, there may be odd diffuse pain which is poorly localized. Unfortunately, the absence of pain is no guarantee of pulpal health and the possible maintenance of vitality.

The visual appearance of the lesion — extent of breakdown, colour of tooth and so on — will provide a valuable indication of its likely depth. This, coupled with the radiographic appearance and the results of vitality tests (Ch. 2), will put the clinician on the right track on the flow chart (Fig. 10.1).

## OPERATIVE TREATMENT

This is best done under rubber dam to reduce the risk of salivary contamination of any exposure to a minimum. The objective is to remove all the peripheral caries, thus obtaining good access to the body of the lesion, and then carefully remove the caries which lies directly over the pulp.

The ideal is to excise the whole lesion, leaving sound dentine as the base of the cavity. However,

DEEP CARIOUS LESION

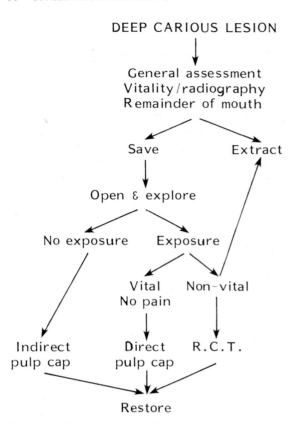

**Fig. 10.1** Management of the deep carious lesion.

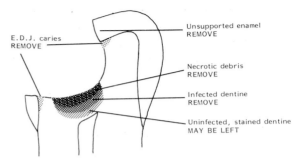

**Fig. 10.2** The zones of a deep carious lesion. EDJ, enamel–dentine junction.

the second, deeper part of the lesion, is only slightly demineralized and contains no bacteria. The structure of the first layer is totally disorganized, whilst the second retains the basic ordered structure of dentine. It is the deeper layer that can be remineralized in favourable conditions (Fig. 10.2).

The application of certain dyes, particularly 1% acid red in propylene glycol solution, stains the superficial, infected layer only, leaving the deeper layer unstained. The dye is applied, washed off and the stained area removed with an excavator. This operation is repeated until the base of the cavity remains unstained. This is a reasonable method of detecting caries, but it must be used with caution. Injudicious or heavy handed removal of the infected tissue may result in a pulpal exposure.

Once the removal of the infected material has been completed, and no exposure has resulted, and if the tooth is restorable, an *indirect pulp cap* is placed. The most reliable material is calcium hydroxide, usually in a resin base, which has two effects. Its high pH of 9–11 will reduce the activity of any bacteria still remaining as the environment changes from acid to alkaline, and also it provokes remineralization of the softened dentine and the deposition of secondary dentine beneath the lesion by the pulp. Since this effect appears to relate to pH, there is some concern about the therapeutic efficacy of recently produced materials which have a pH of 7. However, these new materials do have the advantage of being stronger mechanically and can more readily withstand the occlusal load transmitted via the restoration. The older materials required an extra structural base to absorb this.

when a pulpal exposure might result, it is permissible to leave a zone of altered dentine at the base. It is the identification of the proximity of the pulp and the amount of dentine which may be left, which present the problems. It is very difficult to be sure of the three dimensional relationship of the lesion with the pulp, though, with experience, an educated guess is possible.

In all circumstances, soft, mushy dentine must be removed. However, where there is slight softening, but the dentine appears structurally intact, it is possible to leave this, if the risk of exposure is high. The means of determining the extent of the penetration of the caries are very limited and the use of the conventional dental probe to detect softening could easily lead to penetration of a very thin layer overlying the pulp.

Dyes which are able to differentiate between layers in the dentine may be used. Two layers are important clinically; the first, extensively de-mineralized, contains a large volume of bacteria, and

If the removal of the softened dentine results in an exposure, then the whole lesion should be excised immediately. Contamination of the pulp will have occurred and infected dentine should not remain in the area.

It is now necessary to consider *direct* pulp capping. Again, success depends upon the absence of cellular changes in the pulp, as may be indicated by symptoms. A number of physical criteria also determine the success of the procedure:

1. *Size of the exposure:* the larger the exposure, the less likely is a successful outcome, since contamination of the pulp with infected dentine debris will have occurred. Also haemorrhage will be increased. Ideally the exposure should be less than 0.5 mm in diameter, and one over 1 mm in diameter has a very poor prognosis;

2. *Contamination with saliva:* this will reduce the success rate greatly since there will be bacterial contamination;

3. *Marginal leakage:* any leakage can result in bacterial ingress and direct access to the pulp.

Once the exposure has been located, all the dentine debris should be removed. Any haemorrhage must be arrested, preferably without massive bloodclot formation. Evidence suggests that the presence of a large clot reduces the success rate. The exposure is then treated with calcium hydroxide materials which are free from zinc oxide/eugenol. Again the use of a structural base to prevent displacement of the calcium hydroxide liner is necessary.

Success rate is variable for carious exposures, whilst traumatic exposures are considerably better.

It is, of course, very important to see that there is pulp tissue present. Calcium hydroxide applied to an empty pulp chamber has little value.

*Pulpotomy* may be attempted for large exposures. This involves opening the pulp chamber and amputating the coronal pulp, leaving what is hoped to be healthy pulp in the roots. The root canal pulps are covered with calcium hydroxide.

The success of the procedure depends on the infection being limited to the coronal pulp only, and this will be far from certain. However, if the root canals cannot be negotiated by conventional instruments, pulpotomy gives some hope of retaining the tooth.

**Post-operative assessment**

The patient should be warned of possible pulp symptoms and told to return immediately if there is pain. Regular review using vitality tests and radiographs is essential to ensure that any changes in pathology of the apical tissues may be detected. Calcium hydroxide may cause excessive deposition of secondary dentine which may occlude the root canal. Should this occur, intervention and endodontic therapy may be indicated before the canal is obliterated.

## RESTORATION

In many cases where indirect or direct pulp capping has been necessary, the tooth will have lost a considerable amount of tissue. The plan for restoration should consider, in particular, the retention and stability of the proposed restoration, and the occlusion. Interim temporary dressing should be avoided if possible, since subsequent removal of this and more preparation can insult the pulp further.

Anterior teeth may be restored by pinned or acid-etch retained composite resin, but as will be discussed in Chapter 13, this may have some limitations aesthetically and functionally. Once large amounts of small teeth are lost, then elective devitalization, root filling and a post crown are almost inevitable.

In posterior teeth, where all cusps remain intact, or only a single cusp has been lost, restoration with amalgam is the most reliable solution. Here retention will usually be obtained from the remaining tooth substance and freehand carving will reproduce occlusal stability adequately.

Where more tooth has been lost, then the accurate reproduction of the occlusion will almost certainly require a cast gold crown or inlay. In order to provide a proper foundation for the casting, a core will be necessary.

**Choice of core material**

Three materials may be used for core construction:

• Amalgam
• Composite resin
• Glass ionomer cement

## Amalgam

This has several advantages. It can be well condensed around pins and may be contoured to anatomical form easily. It has good long term durability if crown construction is to be delayed, perhaps whilst oral hygiene is being improved. If there is any dissolution of the cement lute during the life of the crown, corrosion of the amalgam will provide a barrier to leakage.

## Composite resins

These materials are more operator sensitive and appear to have a higher failure rate. They are difficult to adapt around pins and there have been a number of cases of crown failure reported due to separation of the core from the pins.

Unless a specific core building material is used, there will be no colour contrast between it and the tooth. This could make finishing line definition difficult during crown preparation.

## Glass ionomer cements

Currently these materials are of insufficient strength to be used as core materials unless they are supported by a considerable volume of tooth structure. Whilst their therapeutic properties and their dimensional stability are advantages, even the cermet form should not be used except as a fill-in material when cusps remain intact. They can be satisfactory if pins are used with them, but then amalgam has the proven durability.

## Amalgam core placement

Amalgam will always require auxillary retention, though when it is not to be reduced by subsequent crown preparation, careful use of the remaining tooth tissue to provide undercuts can be successful. It is important to remember that any additional aid to retention will weaken the tooth and the dangers of excessive use of pins must be recognized.

The principal means of adding retention are by:

- Pits and grooves
- Pins

## Pits and grooves

The objective is to place the grooves or pits in opposing walls to resist the displacement of the restoration either vertically or laterally. However, their effectiveness can be limited, and they certainly weaken remaining walls. To be of use, any groove must be opposed by another groove or other retentive feature. The two features will then act in concert.

Unless they are of adequate depth, and undercut to allow for the setting contraction of the amalgam, they will serve little purpose. It is also imperative that the amalgam is adequately condensed into them.

## Pins

Pins, whilst aiding retention of the restoration, also introduce planes of weakness in the material and stress concentrations in the tooth. A balance must be established between adequate retention and a restoration that fractures under occlusal stress.

Three types of pin are available:

- Self threading
- Friction grip
- Cemented

**Self threading.** The pinhole is prepared by a twist drill, the diameter of which is slightly smaller than the pin. The pin, usually integral with a bur shank, can then be tapped into place using slow speed. The pin shears off the bur shank as it meets the resistance at the base of the pinhole.

These are the most convenient and safest of the types available, but a number of difficulties can occur during placement:

1. *Oversized pinhole.* This is either the result of the handpiece chuck running eccentrically due to a worn bearing or of lack of positive control of the handpiece as the hole is cut.

2. *Dentine failure.* The speed of rotation or weakness of the dentine can lead to the thread that has been tapped shearing as the pin reaches the bottom of the hole. The pin then comes back with its shank.

3. *Incomplete seating.* This is a particular problem with the self-shearing varieties and can be caused by running the handpiece too fast, or by variations in the elasticity of the dentine resulting in the pin shearing early.

The first two may be corrected by either cutting the next larger hole and trying again with the larger pin, or cementing the pin in place. The latter is difficult, but may be the only solution.

The failure to seat properly may lead to excess pin intruding into the occlusion and also weakness in the support for the pin. If the pin is secure, then it will need bending or cutting. It is better, though, to try to remove it and start again.

Even the successful placement of this type of pin is potentially damaging to the dentine causing crazing and stress concentrations.

*Friction grip.* Here, again, the pinhole is prepared to a slightly smaller size but the pin is pushed home in a holder. This type of pin relies on the elasticity of the dentine to accommodate and retain it, and again there is a risk of stresses and fracture of the dentine under load.

*Cemented.* These pins are cemented into place in slightly oversize holes using low viscosity poly-carboxylate or cyanoacrylate cements. Increased retention may be obtained by sandblasting the pin to produce a mechanical interlock between the dentine, cement and pin. The introduction of the cement into the pinhole may be aided by the use of a spiral root filler.

*Pin placement*

This is particularly important, since the pin must be placed in an area which provides support for the restoration and which does not weaken the tooth. It must also not perforate the pulp or periodontal tissues. There are, therefore, a limited number of sites where pins may be positioned.

Pins should be placed in dentine and to ensure an adequate bulk of dentine surrounding them (Fig. 10.3), they should be about 1 mm inside the enamel–dentine junction. Any closer to the junction, there will be a high risk of fracture of a plate of enamel and dentine away from the side of the tooth. Repair of this, so far below gingival margin level, can be impossible.

The anatomy of the pulp chamber and the interface between the root and the periodontal ligament dictate the angulation of the pin. The pinhole should be parallel to the external root surface and a good guide to this is to place the tip of the bur, or the blade of a flat plastic, in the gingival

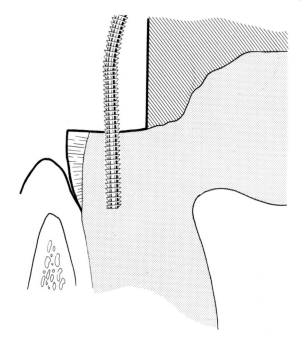

Fig. 10.3 The position of a pin. It should be surrounded by dentine, 1 mm inside the enamel–dentine junction, 2–3 mm deep and bent to fall within the contour of the restoration.

crevice against the root. The bur may then be placed at the same angle on the dentine.

The commencement of the pinhole may be assisted by the cutting of a small depression with a small round bur. The pinhole itself should be cut to a depth of about 2–3 mm, with some brands having a collar fitted to the burs to limit the depth of the hole. The pin should extend the same length above the surface.

After placement, pins should be bent to fall within the contour of the final restoration and sufficient amalgam must overlie the pin so that it does not crack away either during carving or subsequent crown preparation (Fig. 10.4).

Considerable care is necessary during bending since injudicious bending will stress the dentine and cause crazing. A number of devices are available to do this and they work on the principle of gripping the pin just above the point of entry into the dentine. The cemented pins offer the advantage of pre-bending prior to cementation.

Adequate clearance must be obtained between the top of the pin and the surface of the restoration.

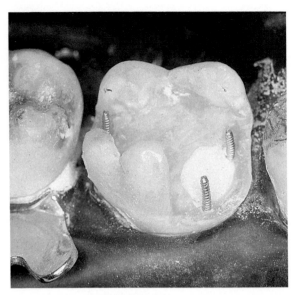

Fig. 10.4 Three pins in place and correctly contoured.

Failure to do this will result in the exposure of the pin either during carving or subsequently during crown preparation.

Reduction of the length of the pin is a dangerous procedure, and the most effective way is to use a diamond in an airturbine. Under no circumstances should a tungsten carbide bur be used as it is likely to fracture. Care should be taken with both self-threading and friction grip pins that they do not start to work loose during this procedure and the patient's pharynx must be protected against swallowing or inhaling the pin.

A rough guide to the number of pins that should be placed is one per cusp lost, with a minimum of two. There should be at least one at each end of a core so that when the occlusal reduction for the crown preparation is done, one section of the core does not drop away (Fig. 10.4).

### Matrices

Placement of matrices on the badly broken down tooth presents a particularly difficult problem. The Siqveland can be very difficult to use since it may ride up the tooth as the band is tightened and slip over the cavity margin, resulting in a negative margin or a space through which amalgam will be exuded. Careful stabilization of the retainer with one hand during packing can help.

The Tofflemire holder with its larger selection of bands may be better and is usually easier to adapt to irregular margins.

However, with both these matrices, the junction where the band enters the retainer can be at an inconvenient point. Under these circumstances, the use of a customized copper band can be useful. This may be trimmed at the chairside, but in the more complex cases an alginate impression may be taken and the band contoured on a stone model. This reduces trauma to the gingival tissue.

Wedging is essential for any matrix so that the band is firmly adapted to the margins of the tooth. Care is necessary to avoid the wedge riding up over the preparation margin (Fig. 9.10).

The establishment of a stable, adequately contoured matrix for a core is vital for the success of this technique.

### Packing and carving

Several successive mixes of amalgam should be used, rather than one large one, since the later ones will be workable at the end of packing.

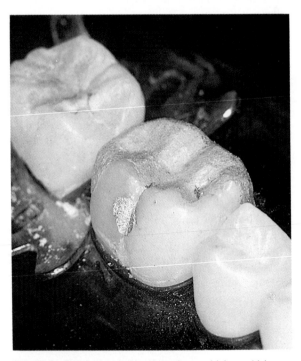

Fig. 10.5 A completed pinned amalgam which would be suitable as a medium term restoration.

In carving a core the aim should be to maintain the contacts with adjacent teeth and stabilize the occlusion. Elaborate anatomical detail is not necessary, provided the crown is to be prepared within a short time. However, if the aim is to produce a medium term restoration, then tooth anatomy should be reproduced to maintain periodontal health (Fig. 10.5).

## SUMMARY

1. Assess pulpal condition as accurately as possible;
2. Remove *all* peripheral caries;
3. Remove pulpal caries with caution and attempt to prevent an exposure;
4. Can the tooth be restored?
5. Indirect pulp cap or direct pulp cap with calcium hydroxide;
6. Provide auxillary retention, usually by pins;
7. Restore with amalgam posteriorly, composite anteriorly;
8. Review pulpal and apical condition regularly.

When constructing the pre-endodontic restoration, it is important not to obstruct access to the root canal(s). If, for example, the whole crown was filled with amalgam, it would be exceedingly tedious and dangerous to find the root canals through this. The roof of the pulp chamber should be overlaid with a weak cement which is easy to remove later.

Anteriorly, if enough coronal dentine is present, a composite resin provisional restoration will be satisfactory. The problems arise if a crown is necessary. A technique that was commonly used was that of a hollow tube temporary post crown, e.g. McGibbon's tube. Whilst superficially attractive, the internal diameter can restrict canal preparation. It is now common practice to make a conventional provisional post crown which is removed at each preparation and filling stage. Of course, this brings complications for rubber dam placement.

## CANAL PREPARATION

### Isolation

Rubber dam is essential, principally to protect the oro-pharynx, and secondarily to minimize contamination of the open root canal. In some areas, it is possible to avoid the use of clamps, which has the advantage that the radiographic appearance is not obscured by metal.

The problem of isolating the crownless root has to be dealt with by using the adjacent teeth for stability, and joining the holes in the dam (Fig. 11.3).

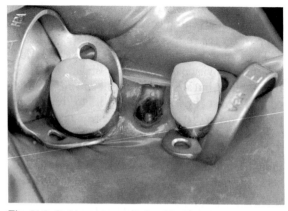

Fig. 11.3 Rubber dam applied to |5 which has had its temporary post crown removed to allow root canal treatment.

### Access

Access must be obtained through the coronal tissues to reach the apical constriction. The preparation of the access cavity must remove the roof of the pulp chamber so that the floor of the chamber and the opening(s) of the root canal(s) can be seen clearly. The access cavity must be placed so that it lies in as near a straight line with the apex as possible, which allows efficient instrumentation with minimum bending of the instruments.

The final breakthrough into the pulp chamber must be done with slow speed, and not the air turbine, to prevent air or water under pressure entering the root canal and passing into the apical tissues. Also, and perhaps more importantly when obtaining access to molars, the roof of the pulp chamber is often very close to the floor, and rapid cutting may perforate the roof, the floor and the furcation. In some circumstances the use of an excavator to remove the roof is a distinct advantage.

Inevitably, the access cavity for a molar will be large, particularly towards the mesial aspect where secondary dentine in the pulp chamber increases the effective root curvature (Fig. 11.4).

There is a compromise between the endodontic

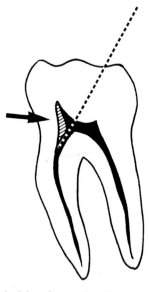

Fig. 11.4 Principles of access in a lower molar. The shaded area of dentine (arrowed) causes the file to become excessively curved. This area of dentine should be removed before the file is inserted.

requirements, where the presence of the crown itself obstructs the root canals, and the restorative requirement, where as much tooth substance as possible should be conserved.

### Pulp extirpation

The barbed broach should be inserted carefully along the canal wall and kept short of the apex to avoid *apical perforation*. To engage the broach in the pulp tissue, it should be twisted and withdrawn in a smooth, gentle action. Sharp movements should be avoided to prevent tearing and incomplete removal. In fine canals, a Hedstroem file of small diameter may be better, since the barbed broach could bind and lodge in the canal.

If the tooth is non-vital, then necrotic tissue should be removed with a file and by irrigation with a 1% sodium hypochlorite solution. The canal must not be prepared in any way before the working distance has been determined.

The problems of obtaining local analgesia for pulp extirpation were discussed in Chapter 3.

### Working distance determination

The position of the apical constriction in relation to a fixed reference point on the crown of the tooth should be determined as accurately as possible, ($\pm$ 0.5 mm). This is essential to ensure correct mechanical preparation which, if short, will leave:

- Necrotic material at the apex
- Untreated pulp space apically

If the working distance is long, the preparation will:

- Destroy the apical constriction
- Damage the apical tissues
- Make filling difficult

The sequence for working distance determination is:

1. Select the largest file that will pass easily into the canal for good radiographic definition;

2. Measure the pre-operative radiograph and compare the root length with average values; decide on the likely working length and set a stop on the file to this length;

3. Note the reference point on the crown (if no crown, use adjacent tooth);

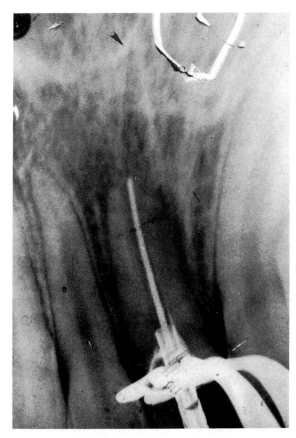

**Fig. 11.5** Periapical diagnostic radiograph with elongation of the apex due to bending of the film in the palate. The apex can just be seen (arrowed) as a faint white line.

4. Insert file slowly; **stop** if obstructed;

5. X-ray (watch for bending of the film and tube angle, Fig. 11.5);

6. Measure the image of the file on the film — it should be $\pm$ 1 mm of reality to indicate minimal distortion; retake if wrong;

7. Measure the distance from the tip of the file to the radiographic apex;

8. If this is greater than 5 mm, increase the insertion of the file, re-X-ray;

9. From an undistorted radiograph, and when the tip of the file is close to the apex, measure the distance from the tip to the apex and add this to the known file length, in millimetres;

10. Subtract 1 mm from the measurement — this is the average position of the apical constriction and is the working distance (Fig. 11.6);

11. Record the distance in the patient's notes.

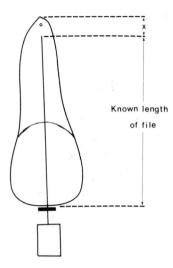

**Fig. 11.6** The determination of the working distance. (X−1) mm is added to the known length of the file, as long as the radiograph is not distorted and X is small.

Mathematical formulae should be avoided since they take no account of unseen curvatures, make no adjustment for hidden radiographic distortions, and errors in measurement are multiplied.

*Electrical conductivity* methods have been proposed, but these are prone to error due to contamination of the canal or in the presence of apical pathology. Recent work has suggested that the error can be as much as 1.5 mm.

### Canal preparation

The preparation must remove infected or degraded dentine, and modify the shape of the pulp space so that it can be filled efficiently.

The optimum shape to receive *laterally condensed and sealed gutta percha* is a smooth walled tube with a continuous taper from the apical constriction to the access cavity. The last 1 mm of the apical region should be of round cross-section to receive the *master cone*.

Perhaps the most important thing to remember during canal preparation is that the canal morphology is extremely variable, and nothing like the rather reassuring image seen on a conventional radiograph. Figure 11. 7 shows a lower incisor X-rayed in the usual labio-lingual view, together with a mesio-distal view. Far from being a conical tube, the canal is irregular, probably has two main branches for

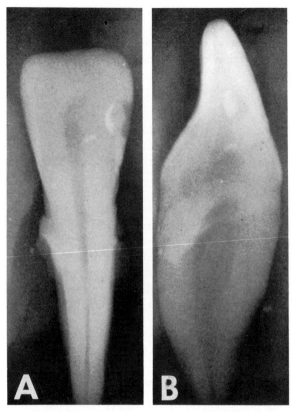

**Fig. 11.7** Radiographs of a lower incisor, showing, **A**, the conventional labio-lingual view and **B**, the 'unknown' shape of the canal when seen from the side.

part of its length, and exhibits sharp curves. In addition, the microscope would reveal connecting branches of pulp, blind and patent lateral canals, and various fin-like projections — none of which can be prepared mechanically. Therefore, all that is prepared are the main, accessible areas, with the hope that the other areas will be sealed and rendered harmless at the filling stage.

The preparation should be done by filing, with copious irrigation with normal saline, and with care to clean debris from both the canal and the files. The danger of using a pure filing action (cutting on the withdrawal stroke) is that debris can be pushed ahead of the file on the upstroke to block the apical region of the canal. Since this is particularly critical in the narrow confines of the last 2–3 mm, the most efficient way to prepare the *apical stop* is to insert the file towards the apex until it binds, either at the working distance or short of it, make a quarter turn to engage the cutting blades with the canal wall and withdraw it completely, bringing the debris out.

When the file reaches the working distance and does not bind, it should be changed to the next file up and the same action continued.

The apical stop should not be enlarged any more when **both**:

- The diameter has reached the minimum size for the material (No. 25 for gutta percha), **and**
- Clean dentine dust has been seen on at least one previous file

The remainder of the canal (that excluding the apical 1 mm) should now be filed circumferentially to flare it outwards towards the crown. It is now unnecessary to twist the file to engage the blades, since pressure can be applied via the handle. The shape will be determined basically by the original canal morphology, and it is necessary to remove an even amount of dentine from its periphery, again until clean dentine dust is brought out and the canal walls offer firm resistance to cutting.

A coarse bladed file, such as the Hedstroem is very efficient for rapid dentine removal. The 'smoother' K-type files are more appropriate for precision in the definition of the apical stop.

The majority of radiographically straight canals have some degree of curve in the apical third. Care must be taken not to create ledges or elbows by trying to take stiff instruments around the bend. The technique to deal with this is to file carefully progressively short of the working distance with progressively larger instruments — the *stepback technique*. Nothing above a No. 35 file will negotiate a curve at the apex, even when pre-curved before insertion in the canal.

The danger of the progressively shortening preparation is the tendency for debris to remain ahead of the files. The working distance must be re-established at each progression by the original apical stop size file, with slight turning to engage and displace the debris.

Canals that are curved in their middle third should be prepared by first cleaning and widening the coronal third to improve access. This may be done by special burs, such as the safe ended Gates-Glidden and then filing the inner aspect of the curve, to 'straighten' the canal within the curved root. The danger here is of filing too much and perforating the inner aspect of the root (Fig. 11.8).

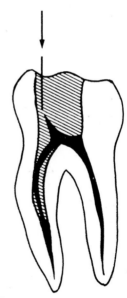

**Fig. 11.8** The preparation of a curved root requires removal of the shaded areas, so that it is effectively straightened.

Ultrasonic filing, oscillating filing and other mechanical systems can be useful, but the principles of the preparation remain the same.

Haemorrhage should not occur during canal preparation. If it does, this may indicate:

- Pulp remnants still present at the apex
- Apical perforation
- Lateral perforation
- Furcation perforation

It will then be necessary to stop, take a radiograph with the apical stop file in place and check the working distance.

Throughout the preparation, irrigation is essential; it:

- Lubricates the files
- Collects debris on the file surface
- Displaces debris

The safest irrigant is normal saline, though 1% sodium hypochlorite is useful as a protein solvent. The needle of the irrigation syringe should not be jammed into the canal, nor should excess pressure be applied when injecting. This would put the apical tissues at risk by fluid accumulation beyond the apex. The excess fluid should be aspirated first and then removed by careful use of paper points. To dry the apical stop, the paper point should be capable of passing close to it (i.e. No. 60 points should not be used in a No. 25 canal).

## MEDICATION

After preparation, canals may be filled by some type of dressing material which could have an anti-microbial effect. Many substances, ranging from antibiotic mixtures to very irritant disinfectants, have been used. No conclusive evidence exists regarding the efficacy of canal medication.

Waiting a week or so between preparation and filling allows any acute apical reaction to pulp extirpation or debris being pushed through the apex to subside without pain. The inflammatory exudate can pass into the partly empty canal.

A mild antimicrobial, with very low irritation is calcium hydroxide in a propylene glycol vehicle. This material is sometimes successful in resolving a persistently oozing canal if left for 4–6 weeks, though replacement is necessary every 10 days or so to maintain activity.

## ROOT FILLING

The tooth to be root filled should:

- Be symptomless
- Not be tender to percussion
- Have no exudate in the root canal(s)

If any of these are present, it indicates continuing pathology. Wash the canal to remove the dressing, dry it, re-establish the working distance with the apical stop file and re-dress. Review in 7–10 days.

The canal should be filled with a material impervious to tissue fluid, which prevents leakage between itself and the canal walls, and seals off all communication between the pulp space and the periodontal ligament.

A wide range of materials, from metal cones to polypharmaceutical pastes is available, most having a reasonable success rate. Currently the most acceptable materials are gutta percha (GP) with sealing cement, coupled with silver cones in very curved, fine canals.

Both GP and silver techniques require that a *master cone* reaches the apical stop and fits the terminal zone of the preparation accurately. The master cone must match the file size as closely as possible, but some variation in the GP cones is inevitable because of difficulties in manufacture.

Silver is appropriate for canals prepared to less than 25 because of curves or obstructions; GP is appropriate for the rest.

Most *root sealing materials* are ZOE based with additives for radio-opacity, disinfection and inflammation reduction. Care is important in the choice of material in case any passes beyond the apex. Paraformaldehyde containing materials cannot be recommended, for this reason.

After placement of the master cone, *lateral* or *accessory cones* are condensed into place together with the sealer. This means that the working time of the sealer should be sufficiently long to allow this.

The sequence for root filling is:

1. Remove the dressing from the canal, re-establish the apical stop with the appropriate file;
2. Select the GP point of the apical stop size and mark the working distance on it; insert it into the canal slowly;
3. Make sure the point reaches the working distance and is a good fit ('tug back');
4. X-ray to check that the GP fits to the working distance. If the point does not fit to the working distance when tried in, or is short when X-rayed, repeat the preparation of the apical stop to either clear debris, or extend the preparation if it is short. Re-check the diameter of the GP point on gauge, and if necessary, try another one of the same nominal size. The GP try-in also checks the preparation in addition to checking the master cone fit.

Then:

5. Mix sealer and place a range of accessory cones with their tips in the sealer;
6. Select a file size smaller than the apical stop and coat this with sealer and, with an anticlockwise rotation, coat the canal walls with sealer, up to the stop;
7. Coat the master cone with sealer, insert it carefully (beware hydraulic effects of pain, or extrusion) to the marked working distance;
8. Using lateral spreaders, beginning with the smallest, make room for accessory cones alongside the master cone and build up the full filling sequentially;

9. Take a post-operative radiograph and seal the access cavity. If the canal is *overfilled*, tell the patient and keep it under review. If the canal is *underfilled*, because of technical error, remove the root filling and start again. If this underfill goes to the working distance which is short because of some obstruction, then again tell the patient, and keep it under review.

### Open apex

This may occur as a result of incomplete root formation (Ch. 3) or because of instrumentation beyond the apical constriction (apical perforation). It makes root filling difficult because there is no restriction to the escape of sealer into the apical tissues. In the immature root, the canal is funnel shaped, becoming wider towards the apex. Conventional condensation is then almost impossible.

The preparation of the immature canal should be done by careful circumferential filing, since the apical diameter is usually larger than the largest file. The root filling should be made up, by trial and error, by warming and coalescing several GP points into a large single cone of the right diameter. This can be tried-in in the usual way and then sealed carefully, avoiding extrusion into the tissues.

Filling a canal with an apical perforation is also difficult. The length of insertion of the master cone must be controlled carefully, and it should be held against the crown while inserting lateral cones, so that the spreaders do not push it past the apex. Lateral condensation must be gentle, to avoid extrusion of sealer.

### REVIEW

Apical tissues take time to heal, and progress should be monitored radiographically at six months after filling, a year after that, and then every two or three years. There is an incidence of recurrent infection around apparently successful root fillings which may relate to lateral canals, or to short zones of unfilled apical canal.

Healing of the root end is by the laying down of cementum across the apical foramen and possibly the presence of clean dentine dust will help this. There may be a very small zone of dentine chippings at the final extent of successful root fillings.

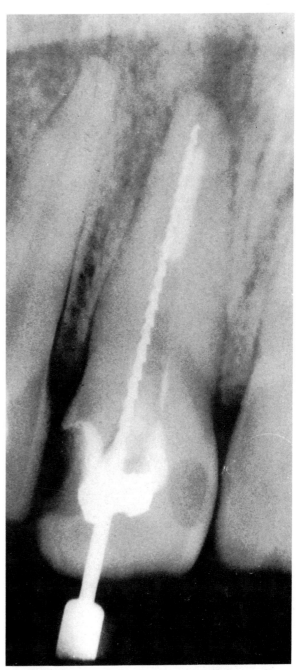

**Fig 11.9**  The removal of a GP point with a Hedstroem file. This file is ideal because of its rearward facing barbs.

### RECURRENT INFECTION

Symptoms, or radiographic appearance of an increasing area of radiolucency at the apex indicate pathology and failure of the root filling. Either:

- Removal and repreparation of the root filling (Fig. 11.9)
- Endodontic surgery

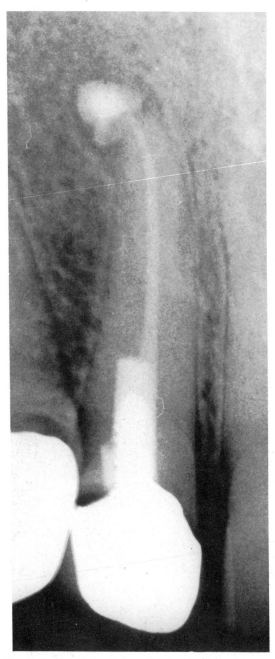

**Fig 11.10**  Extruded sealer associated with a long standing and static apical area at ⎣2⎦. No treatment is required for this. The crown needs replacing though.

Intervention should not be made in cases of long standing, symptomless over- or under-filled canals (Fig. 11.10), though there could be an exception to this if the tooth was to receive a crown or be a bridge abutment.

## ENDODONTIC SURGERY

The surgical approach to the root apex is required to place an apical seal when the conventional approach through the root is impossible, or when an apparently well executed root filling has failed. Surgery should be reserved for these cases and should not be used to correct symptomless and signless filling errors.

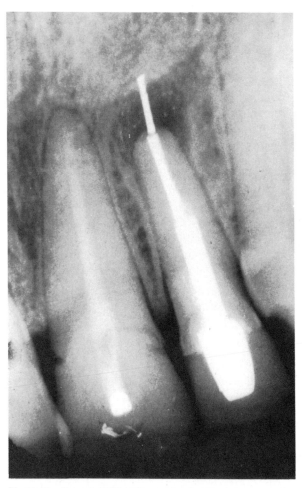

**Fig 11.11**  Extruded GP in ⎣2 associated with symptoms and a sinus. There is a very good post crown present, and the extruded filling probably could not be retrieved anyway. The tooth was apicected. The post-operative radiographs are shown in Figures 3.4 and 3.5.

The circumstances in which to consider surgery are, in the *presence of infection*, canals that are non-negotiable because of:

- Secondary dentine, curves, pulp stones
- Fractured instruments
- Post crowns (Fig. 11.11)
- Unremovable root fillings

or canals that are difficult to fill because of:

- Lateral canals
- An open apex

Surgery may also be used to provide treatment rapidly, or to deal with infection that persists in spite of repeated dressing.

If the unremovable root filling is an apical silver point or a retrograde amalgam, and the remainder of the canal is empty, then the cause of the infection may be leakage past the filling into the canal. Bacteria can obtain their nutrient from the leakage and toxins pass out into the tissues. In this case it is worth trying to prepare the empty canal and fill it up to the existing root filling (Fig. 11.12).

### Apicectomy technique

Local analgesia is usually acceptable for most single teeth. General anaesthesia may be indicated for several teeth or apprehensive individuals. The analgesia must be effective, with palatal and incisive canal blocks being necessary for upper anterior teeth.

The sequence is:

1. Analgesia;
2. Raise full gingival flap with bevelled incision at the papillae (Fig. 11.13); this gives good access and little scarring;

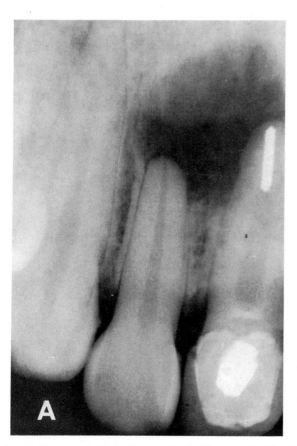
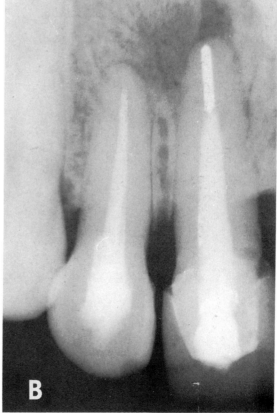

**Fig. 11.12**  **A**, Apical infection associated with a non-vital 2| and an apical silver point in 1|. This was treated by conventional root canal therapy of 2| and root filling the 1| up to the silver. **B**, The result was complete resolution of the infection without surgery.

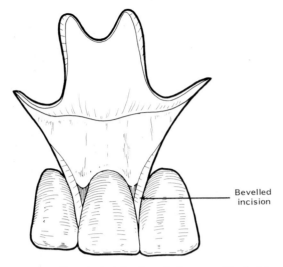

Bevelled incision

**Fig. 11.13** Full gingival flap for apical surgery. The incision at the gingival papillae is bevelled to provide a broad area for replacement, which reduces recession.

3. Identify the apical region by pressure with an excavator to try perforating the cortical plate over the infected area. Otherwise, measure the root length from the pre-operative radiograph;

4. Remove cortical bone with slow speed burs with copious irrigation;

5. Avoid scarring the root by working higher than the apical level initially;

6. Obtain clear access to the root apex and identify any anatomical structures of relevance, e.g. antrum, mental nerve;

7. Clear any soft tissue around the apex — excision biopsy;

8. Reduce the apex by a bevelled cut, so that the root face is angled towards the operator;

9. Cut a 2–3 mm deep undercut cavity in the root canal end;

10. Wash, dry, and pack the bone with ribbon gauze to isolate the apex;

11. Place retrograde amalgam;

12. Remove gauze and excess amalgam, irrigate, close and suture.

Systemic antibiotics should be prescribed pre-operatively for medical problems, or post-operatively for the prevention of infection in a large bony cavity.

The more posterior the tooth, the more difficult will be the surgery and the more likely there will be anatomical complications.

The palatal roots of upper premolars are difficult to reach and see. Palatal roots of upper molars are impossible to reach and see, but these are straight and can usually be root filled conventionally. The buccal roots are easily accessible by surgery.

The maxillary antrum lies close to the upper premolars and molars. Antral perforation does not usually give rise to problems because the flap closes it. The patient should be given systemic antibiotics and told not to blow his nose.

The mental nerve is a complication of lower premolars, and the hazard of mental anaesthesia must be mentioned when consent to apicectomy in the region is sought.

The inferior dental nerve is close to the lower molars and these should not be apicected.

Finally, a retrograde amalgam must always be placed, rather than relying on the sealing ability of the existing root filling, which may be disturbed when cut.

Where a post crown is to placed, make the post before the surgery in case the preparation of the post displaces the apical seal if the retrograde amalgam is already there (Fig. 11.14).

Apical bone may take several months, sometimes over a year, to fill in. This should be monitored radiographically at regular review (Figs. 3.4 and 3.5).

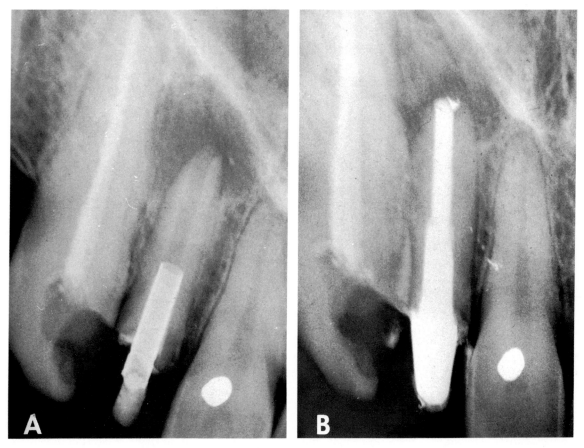

**Fig. 11.14   A,** The 2| has an open apex and a persistent apical area. Dressing with calcium hydroxide through a McGibbon's tube has been unsuccessful. **B,** A long post has been inserted in 2| prior to the placement of the retrograde amalgam. A provisional crown is placed at the same time to wait for gingival healing.

# 12. Principles of occlusal management

*P. H. Jacobsen*

The functional anatomy of the occlusion was described in Chapter 7. This chapter discusses the clinical techniques associated with the occlusion, particularly the use of articulators.

## EQUIPMENT

The equipment available for occlusal management ranges from the primitive to the esoteric, from bare hands to microcomputers. The very simple articulators, the average path and simple plane line, do not locate any hinge axis from the patient and cannot receive pre-centric records effectively. At the other end of the scale, the computerized, fully adjustable articulator will provide the nearest equivalent to the patient, with curved condylar guides, immediate and progressive side-shifts, exact inter-condylar width and the true hinge axis.

The overriding consideration in the choice of equipment is to use that which is appropriate to the job in hand, and that both the dentist and the technician really know and understand the principles of the instruments they use. A badly used articulator is often much, much worse than no articulator at all.

Incorrect mounting will lead to restorations which will require considerable chairside time for fitting, whilst the occlusal surfaces are modified to suit the actual occlusion.

The most practical type of instrument is the semi-adjustable articulator and its associated face-bow. There are several excellent types available and the choice depends to a large extent on personal preference. This book shows cases mounted on the Dentatus ARH and the Whipmix 8300. The first tends to be used extensively in dental schools in prosthetics, and the latter is a light, simple instrument which is more suitable for conservative dentistry.

In order to illustrate the design of face-bows and articulators, the Whipmix 8300 will be described in detail.

## Face-bow

The purpose of the face-bow is to orientate the upper model in three planes to the condylar assembly. The majority operate in connection with an arbitrary hinge axis, which is used to make the recording easier.

A number of workers have derived positions for the abitrary hinge axis by approximating the location of the true hinge axis, and these are usually claimed to be within 5 mm of the true axis on all patients. The most common is a point 12 mm anterior to the posterior border of the tragus along a line drawn from the superior border of the tragus to the outer canthus of the eye. This position would be translated by a face-bow to the condylar axis of the articulator.

However, it is easier to use an ear-bow (Fig. 12.1) which locates into the external auditory meatus, with the articulator having mounting sites to receive this bow and derive the arbitrary axis (Fig. 12.2).

The Whipmix ear-bow (Fig. 12.1) is a self-centering bow which can also measure the inter-condylar distance. The bow is located in the vertical plane by the bridge of the nose. The bite fork should locate the upper model accurately, but without engaging tooth undercut to avoid distortion. Three layers of base plate wax, softened and firmly sealed to the metal are sufficient, and a ZOE wash can be added for extra accuracy if required.

In taking the record, it should be ensured that:

1. The ear lugs are firmly engaged on bone;
2. The bridge of nose is firmly engaged by the bridge piece;

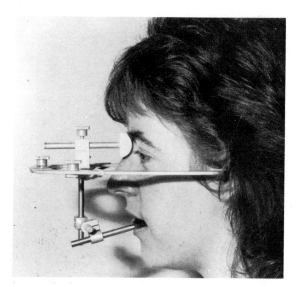

**Fig. 12.1** The Whipmix ear-bow in place. The bow is self-centering and locates to the bridge of the nose for its vertical reference point.

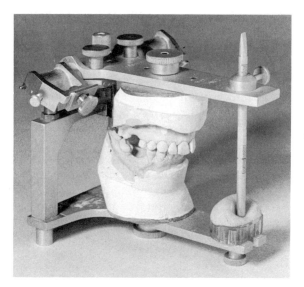

**Fig. 12.3** The Whipmix 8300 articulator. This is a light Arcon instrument, with adjustable condylar angles and immediate side-shift. The progressive side-shift is fixed.

## Articulator

The Whipmix 8300 (Fig. 12.3) is a simple, light 'Arcon' type semi-adjustable articulator. The 'Arcon' classification describes the fact that the

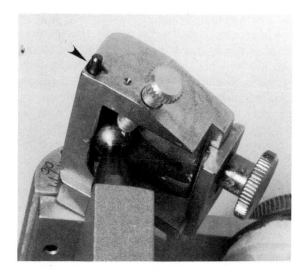

**Fig. 12.2** The ear-bow mounting point on the Whipmix 8300 articulator (arrowed). This point is 12 mm posterior to the condylar axis and therefore reproduces an arbitrary hinge axis.

3. The bite fork is accurately and evenly located on all the teeth and stabilized either by the clinician or the patient during recording;
4. All screws etc, are tightened very firmly.

It is useful to have the articulator at the chairside to check the ear-bow settings and discover spurious recordings whilst the patient is still available.

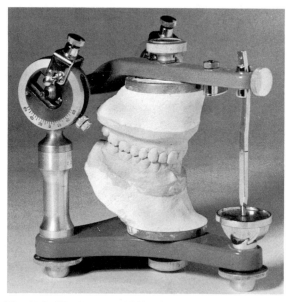

**Fig. 12.4** The Dentatus ARH articulator. This is a non-Arcon instrument, with adjustable condylar angles and progressive side-shift. It has no provision for immediate side-shift.

condyles are attached to the lower member in comparison with the Dentatus ARH which is 'non-Arcon', having the condyles on the upper member (Fig. 12.4).

The Arcon design is more realistic anatomically, since in protrusion the condyles move forward with the mandible. In the non-Arcon, the condyles move backwards. Some minor technical advantages are also claimed for the Arcon type.

The Whipmix can be set to vary the condylar angles and the immediate side-shift. Its progressive side-shift is fixed, as is its intercondylar distance. It has curved condylar pathways and the incisal guide can be customized to the anterior guidance (p. 117).

## Occlusal records

There are three types of static occlusal records, each for a different purpose. In addition, dynamic records can be used for certain articulators.

### Pre-centric record

This is a tooth-apart record, taken with the patient on the retruded arc of closure. It is used to carry out a *pre-operative occlusal analysis* where problems have been diagnosed with the existing centric occlusion.

### Centric record

This is a tooth-together record of the position of maximum intercuspation. This position would be used for mounting pre-operative and master models when no change to the existing centric occlusion is proposed. However, the best way of orientating the models is to avoid the use of an inter-dental record altogether, and place them into the position of 'best fit'. This position can be checked against the patient and marked on the models.

### Lateral and protrusive check records

These are used to set the articulator condylar angles and the instruction manual of the articulator will specify those required for a particular instrument.

### Dynamic records

A detailed description of these is outside the scope of this book. Basically, these are usually tracings or microcomputer signals from specialized face-bow systems.

They can be used to:

- Assess the amount of immediate and progressive side-shift
- Assess the condylar inclination
- Trace the condylar path shape
- Trace the incisal guide
- Trace the chewing cycle
- Assess muscle activity and functional disturbances

### Recording media

The essential requirements are that the recording medium should not interfere with the path of closure of the mandible, should record sufficient detail accurately to permit orientation of the models and be sufficiently rigid to stabilize the models during mounting on the articulator.

The commonly used wax squash bite has the major disadvantage of interfering with the path of closure and also obscure the tooth position that is being recorded. Softer materials, such as alginate and impression rubbers, have been used to overcome this problem, but they give imprecise mounting positions for the models during articulation.

The technique to be described for a pre-centric record offers rigidity and the minimum interference with closure. The starting point is accurate study models, taken in an elastomer and cast with die stone occlusal surfaces. The record consists of two thicknesses of very hard baseplate wax supported by a metal mesh. The mesh is cut to fit exactly to the palatal surfaces of the upper teeth and the wax is trimmed to the buccal surfaces (Figs 12.5 and 12.6). This ensures good vision of the tooth relationships.

Bimanual manipulation of the mandible onto the hinge axis is now performed. The patient is asked to half open the mouth and relax. The operator's fingers and thumbs exert upwards and backwards pressure on the mandible to locate the condyles into the glenoid fossae on the hinge axis (Fig. 12.7).

The wax wafer is softened in hot water and placed on the upper arch and the mandible manipulated on the hinge axis so that the lower teeth indent the wax by about 0.5 mm. The wafer is removed and chilled

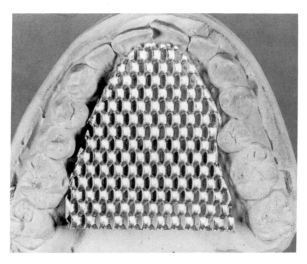

**Fig. 12.5** Occlusal record. Expanded metal mesh cut to fit to the palatal aspect of the upper arch. The mesh supports the recording wax.

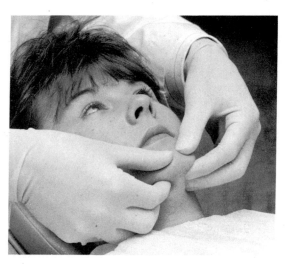

**Fig. 12.7** Manipulation on to the retruded arc of closure. The operator's fingers and thumbs exert upward and backward pressure to locate the condyles into their most superior, posterior position and rotate the mandible.

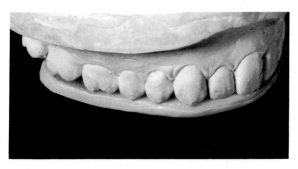

**Fig. 12.6** Two thicknesses of hard wax have been added to sandwich the mesh. The wax is trimmed to the buccal surfaces so that the occlusal relationship can be seen during the registration.

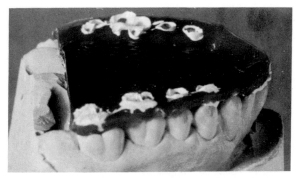

**Fig. 12.8** Pre-centric record tried on the upper model. The ZOE wash should fit accurately to the cusp tips. The upper surface of the record shows the reproduction of the lower arch cusp tips and no other detail.

in cold water. The detail of the tooth relationship can now be recorded using a zinc oxide–eugenol wash. The wash is 'dotted' into the tooth indents on both surfaces of the wax with just enough used to record the cusp tips only. Any more may record occlusal surface detail not included on the models and therefore prevent seating of the record. The wafer is replaced in the mouth and the mandible manipulated again on the hinge axis. The record is removed and carefully placed on each model in turn to check for accurate seating. This checks the accuracy of both the record and the models (Fig. 12.8).

To confirm the reproducibility of the record, two further wafers can be taken and the mounting done by a split cast technique. Here, the upper model is grooved and a separating medium applied. It is mounted to the face-bow in the usual way, and the lower model plastered to the first record. When the plaster has set, the record is removed and the upper model separated from its mounting plaster leaving the locating points. The other two records are then used to orientate the upper model onto the mounted lower model, and the articulator closed. If the records are identical, then the location grooves and points will meet exactly. Two out of three is an acceptable reproduction.

In the case of resistant patients, a 'deprogrammer' may be needed to remove the memory of CO. The

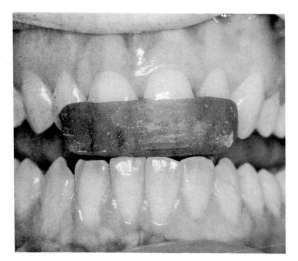

**Fig. 12.9** An occlusal deprogrammer. This removes the memory of centric occlusion and, after removal, manipulation onto the retruded arc of closure should be easier.

appliance is made at the chairside from cold-cure acrylic and forms a flat bite plane on the incisal edges (Fig. 12.9). The record is reattempted after about ten minutes, with the deprogrammer out.

The same wax wafer arrangement may be used for lateral and protrusive records for articulator settings in accordance with the manufacturer's directions. The Whipmix can also be set by the simple recording

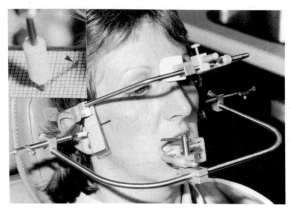

**Fig. 12.10** A simple dynamic recording device which registers the condylar path. The lower bar is attached to the lower incisors, and the teeth are discluded so that the mandible can be freely protruded. The condylar angle is read from the trace (left trace inset, arrow indicates the true hinge axis). The instrument also demonstrates any immediate side-shift.

device shown in Figure 12.10. This traces the condylar path and indicates the immediate side-shift.

## OCCLUSAL ANALYSIS

This can only be done by clinical examination, but the procedure is aided by having an accurate articulator mounting to hand.

### Clinical examination of the occlusion

*General visual examination*

This will form part of the full examination of the patient as described in Chapter 2. The following aspects are of particular interest with regard to the occlusion:

- Missing teeth or malposed teeth
- Cuspal height and cuspal inclines
- Curves of Spee and Monson, incisal inclination
- Tooth surfaces — wear facets, irregular loss, attrition, erosion and abrasion
- Restorations/prostheses — particularly occlusal form and function
- Centric occlusion, overbite, overjet, crossbite
- Centric relation and the retruded arc of closure

*Detailed examination*

This may be done alongside an articulation to confirm it, or as a clinical procedure only. The exercise requires 8 μm metal foil (shimstock) and

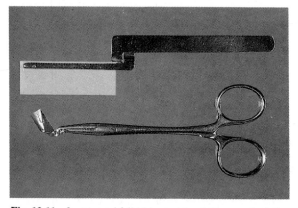

**Fig. 12.11** 8 μm metal foil (shimstock) and 40 μm articulating paper.

artery forceps, 40 μm smudge-proof articulating paper, red and blue, with reverse action tweezers (Fig. 12.11).

The shimstock is used to check the existence of stable, contacting cusp/fossa relationships. The patient should be asked to close until the teeth are just touching, since variable compression of the periodontal ligaments can bring uneven or open sites into contact. This point is of considerable importance when fitting restorations since clenching can create apparent evenness of contacts. Shimstock is placed between each area of likely contact, the patient closes, and the foil will either be held or pull out (Fig. 12.12). This can be noted and checked against the articulation later.

Next, use blue paper to mark centric occlusion contacts. The teeth should be dried and the patient asked to close the teeth together. A variety of markings are possible, from the classic tripod, to single fossa contacts (Fig. 12.13). Red paper is now used to demonstrate precentric prematurities. The patient is manipulated onto the hinge axis and closed into the retruded contact position. Then he closes of his own volition into centric occlusion. The markings of red and blue will either be superimposed, in which case they are the centric stops, or the red will be isolated. The isolated red markings are the premature

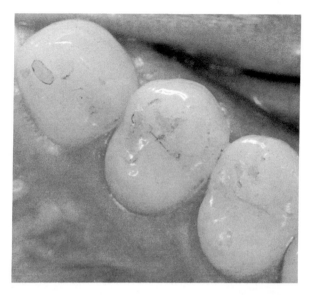

**Fig. 12.13** Centric occlusion contacts shown by articulating paper. The single centric stop contact from the lower canine shows as the major mark on the upper canine. The upper first premolar receives the supporting cusp from the lower first premolar as a tripod contact in its mesial fossa.

contacts and the slide pathway should be red, leading into red superimposed on blue (Fig. 12.14).

Examination of lateral and protrusive excursions should demonstrate either canine guidance or group function, and the length and height of the anterior guidance. This latter characteristic is shown by the amount of posterior disclusion (Ch. 7).

The most important aspect of the eccentric excursions is to look for *non-working interferences*. Classically, on lateral excursion, the second molars of the non-working side may be in contact (Fig. 12.15). This is considered to be a departure from occlusal norms and might be a predisposing factor in TMJ dysfunction. The 'proper' relationship is that the

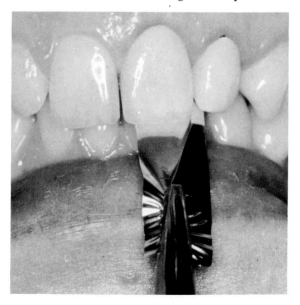

**Fig. 12.12** Shimstock being used to check the centric contact between the upper and lower central incisors.

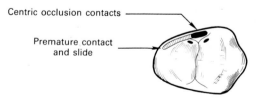

Centric occlusion contacts

Premature contact and slide

**Fig. 12.14** Diagram of a typical pre-centric prematurity on an upper premolar. The lower supporting cusp meets the mesial incline of the palatal cusp and slides up that incline to reach a tripod fossa contact in centric occlusion.

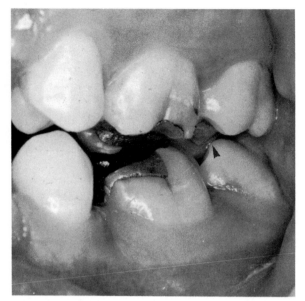

Fig. 12.15 Non-working interference between the upper and lower second molars (arrowed).

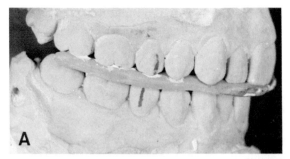

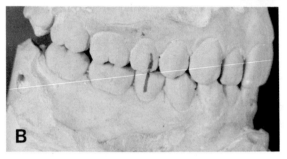

Fig. 12.16 **A**, Articulated models with pre-centric record in place; **B**, The record has been removed and the articulator closed. There has been an upward and forward movement, as shown by the marks on the premolars, to reach centric occlusion.

mandible should have tooth guidance on the working side, but only condylar guidance on the non-working side.

### Confirmation of articulated mounting

The articulation should be compared with the patient. This will involve the use of articulating paper and shimstock and general observation of the tooth relationships created by articulator movements.

When the pre-centric record is removed, the articulator should reproduce the retruded arc of closure, with the retruded contact position and then close into centric occlusion via sliding from the prematurities (Fig. 12.16). In CO, shimstock should be retained by centric stops on the articulator as it is in the mouth (Fig. 12.17). Wear facets should be observed in particular, to see that these approximate to each other on the models as they do clinically.

Comparison of the articulating paper markings made clinically in CO, retruded contact position and in eccentric excursions with those on the articulator should show good agreement.

### Errors in articulation

These can occur as a result of the compromises made

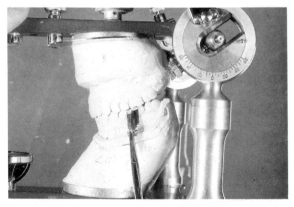

Fig. 12.17 The centric occlusion contacts on the articulator being checked with shimstock.

in articulator design and particularly as a result of using an arbitrary hinge axis. It may be possible to compensate for some errors by adjusting the condylar assemblies to bring appropriate teeth into contact, but gross inaccuracies will require remounting to a new occlusal record.

Possible sources of error in articulation are:

1. Distortion of the impression;
2. Air blows on the occlusal surface;
3. Slippage of the face-bow;
4. Use of the arbitrary hinge axis;
5. Expansion of the mounting plaster;
6. Incorrect centric record;
7. Articulator design compromises;
8. Compression of the periodontium not reproduced;
9. Incorrect angles set.

## OCCLUSAL EQUILIBRATION

This procedure, sometimes referred to as 'selective grinding', involves the recontouring of tooth surfaces so that the occlusion conforms to certain norms. The indications are contentious and there is much disagreement on whether the procedure should be performed. Various workers have proposed occlusal equilibration in the following circumstances:

1. The attainment of occlusal harmony for all patients as a preventive measure;
2. As part of periodontal therapy;
3. Treatment for TMJ dysfunction syndrome;
4. Pre-operative mouth preparation for crown and bridgework.

The doctrinaire 'equilibration for all' is not indicated by the available evidence, which suggests that almost all people have occlusal interferences but only a small proportion are suffering from an occlusal related disorder (Ch. 20). The use of equilibration for an established disorder is also considered later.

The occlusal aetiological component in periodontal disease is currently discredited. Studies in Scandinavia have suggested that occlusal forces are regulated by a feedback mechanism which relates them to the amount of support available.

However, there is some evidence that limited equilibration is of value prior to crown and bridge-work. The preparations will remove occlusal surface and, in doing so, may remove existing prematurities. This will change the tooth guidance and may also change the CO position. The practical result might be the loss of occlusal clearance when the restoration is tried in. If the second molar shown in Figure 12.15 were reduced, then the condylar guidance would take over the pathway and no crown could fit in between.

## Technique

Equilibration must be approached with extreme care — the enamel cannot be put back. Further, the removal of apparently simple and localized prematurities can have the knock-on effect of creating more elsewhere. The experienced operator can adjust an occlusion using the clinical marking technique described earlier, but the tyro is advised to try out this scheme on an articulator first. Large texts on 'occlusion' may be read to provide details of doctrinaire approaches, but this chapter will deal with the simple correction of prematurities and interferences.

The basic concept is to allow closure on multiple arcs of closure into a CO position that has a range of 1 mm or so both antero-posteriorly and bucco-lingually — a true long centric. The attainment of any position within long centric can then be achieved without the intrusion of premature contacts.

In lateral movements, all teeth on the non-working side should be discluded, as should all palatal cusps on the working side. In protrusion, all the posterior teeth should disclude, and the lower anterior teeth should have even and balanced contact with the upper teeth.

The following rules should be applied:

1. Do not reduce the height of any supporting cusps;
2. Fossae may be widened but must not be deepened;
3. Prematurities and interferences should be removed by hollowing cusp slopes;
4. Non-supporting cusps can be reduced in height to remove non-working interferences.

These rules are illustrated in the series of diagrams in Figure 12.18.

## RESTORATIVE IMPLICATIONS

As has already been stated, each individual adapts successfully to his occlusal irregularities, and can continue adapting as teeth are lost or restored. However, there must clearly be a limit to the capacity of this adaptation and so the golden rule of occlusal restoration is not to create further problems.

This principle is enshrined in the 'conformative' approach to occlusal restoration. Where centric occlusion and its associated lateral and protrusive

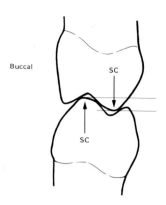

**Buccal**

SC

SC

**A**

**Fig. 12.18** Principles of occlusal equilibration, assuming a correct and stable CO. **A**, CO. The contacts between the pairs of centric stops and supporting cusps must be maintained for occlusal stability.

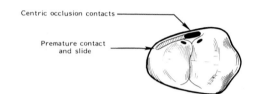

Centric occlusion contacts

Premature contact and slide

**B**

**B**, Precentric prematurity on an upper premolar. Hollow the mesial slope of the palatal cusp, but do not touch the tripod contacts where the two articulating paper colours will be superimposed from CO.

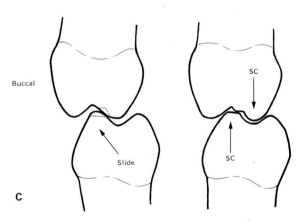

Buccal

SC

SC

SC

Slide

**C**

**C**, Lateral slide from a pre-centric prematurity between the palatal cusp of the upper molar and the buccal cusp of the lower molar. The mandible moves to the right after this contact, into CO. Widen the fossa on the upper, but keep its contact level the same. Reduce the tip of the buccal cusp of the lower, maintaining the same buccal inclined plane contact, and creating a new plateau contact for stability to the palatal aspect.

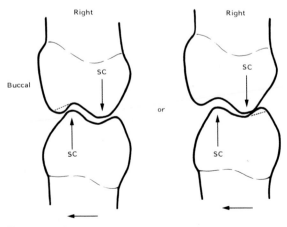

Right

Right

SC

SC

Buccal

or

SC

SC

**D**

Direction of movement to right working side

**D**, Working side interferences: grind non-supporting cusps i.e. buccal upper, lingual lower, depending on the excursion. The interferences shown will tend to occur only in group function, since canine guidance tends to disclude all the posterior teeth. The adjustment will balance the excursion.

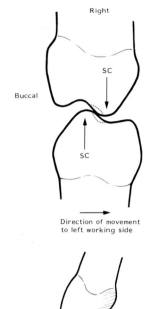

E

**E**, Non-working interferences. Hollow the cusp slopes of interfering inclines, without removing cusp tips.

F

**F**, Protrusive interference. Ideally, the lower incisors should have an even path and contacts with the uppers. The diagram shows the adjustment required if the lower incisor has an isolated path, discluding the others. The lower incisor tip must not be reduced — it would then be out of contact in centric, and would overerupt.

movements are functioning satisfactorily, then no procedure must interfere with this. No doctrinaire philosophies of the rights or wrongs of a particular occlusion should intrude on treatment. Each new restoration should blend harmoniously with the functional pattern already present, provided that is satisfactory.

## Occlusal stability

The maintenance of a stable CO position is important for occlusal harmony. This may be influenced by restorative work and the behaviour of materials.

### Intracoronal restorations

As was mentioned earlier, the natural cusp/fossa relationship is very difficult to reproduce by freehand carving. The result of inaccurate contacts, or no contacts at all, will be tooth movement to seek a stable position (Fig. 12.19).

In moderate to large restorations, the natural fossa

should be replaced by a flat plateau (Fig. 12.20), which receives the supporting cusp of the opposing tooth. This provides good stability and also directs

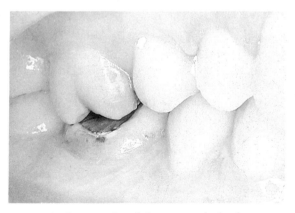

**Fig. 12.19** Over-eruption of the upper molar has been caused by poor reproduction of the occlusal surface of its opponent. To correct this, the upper occlusal plane must be re-aligned by adjusting the displaced molar, or crowning it, followed by a veneer crown on the lower to maintain the new position.

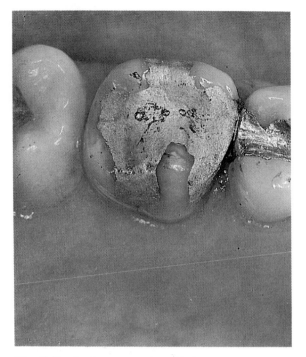

**Fig. 12.20**   Amalgam restoration with flat plateaux centric stops.

the occlusal loads axially. However, the best restoration from the occlusal viewpoint is the small one. Absolutely minimal cutting of the occlusal surface will allow the occlusion to be maintained by enamel in its original state (Fig. 9.2).

### Choice of materials

The choice of materials to restore occlusal surfaces is equally important. No wholly satisfactory material exists; all direct restorative materials deform under load or undergo surface loss and, of the indirect materials, ceramic is the most difficult to use efficiently. Table 12.1 summarizes factors which

**Table 12.1**   Factors involved in the selection of materials for occlusal surfaces

| Metal | Ceramic |
|---|---|
| Large pulps | Small pulps |
| Small teeth | Large teeth |
| Low anterior guidance | High anterior guidance |
| Average technical support | Excellent technical support |
| Simple clinical adjustment | Difficult clinical adjustment |

influence the choice between cast metal and ceramic for the restoration of occlusal surfaces.

The relationship of preparations to pulpal and tooth size will be discussed in Chapter 13.

A low anterior guidance leads to very little posterior disclusion and therefore the occlusal clearance required to accommodate ceramic may result in a very short preparation. A larger posterior disclusion will permit ceramic coverage.

The average technician is usually skilled in handling wax and will be able to generate a functional surface in metal very adequately. However, when firing ceramic it is much more difficult to achieve accurate contacts.

Perhaps the most important veto is provided by the last factor in Table 12.1. Marking, adjustment and repolishing of metal is much less time-consuming clinically than the procedure for ceramic, which should include reglazing. Unless aesthetics are of overriding importance, the better material for occlusal surfaces is cast metal (Fig. 12.21).

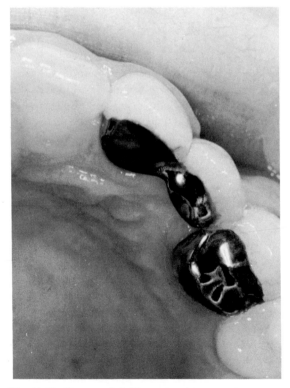

**Fig. 12.21**   Upper arch bridgework, with most of the functional surfaces reproduced in metal.

## Bridgework

It is essential that bridgework replaces all the functional contacts in centric occlusion. It used to be suggested that loads on the abutment teeth could be reduced by narrowing the occlusal table of the pontics. This is questionable, but more importantly such a pontic may not have correct centric contacts.

Figure 12.22 shows a case where occlusal contacts were not provided, leading to considerable problems. The patient was a 45-year-old man, who was complaining that the gap between the lower left lateral incisor and the canine was opening progressively (Fig. 12.22A). This, in fact was caused by overeruption of the canine, and the bridge pontic opposing this tooth (Fig. 12.22B) had no centric stop. Orthodontic therapy was provided to realign the

canine (Fig. 12.22C), and the upper bridge was remade with a positive fossa relationship with the repositioned tooth. This took almost two years.

## Anterior guidance

The functional contours of upper anterior teeth are particularly important, and when making crowns or bridges for that region, the articulator must be 'customized' to reproduce conformative movement pathways. This is done at the diagnostic mounting stage and either an adjustable incisal guide can be set to the appropriate angles or, for better accuracy, a customized incisal table can be made (Fig. 12.23).

Cold curing acrylic is added to the incisal table, and whilst it is soft, the articulator is moved through the

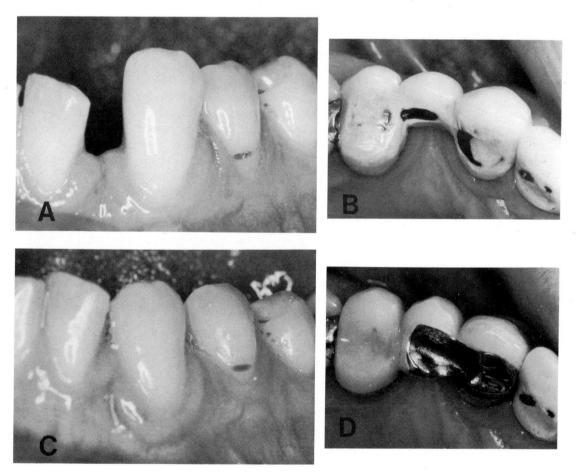

**Fig. 12.22** Loss of occlusal stability. The lower canine has overerupted (**A**) because there is no centric stop on the upper bridge pontic (**B**). The tooth was realigned orthodontically (**C**), and a new bridge made with a positive centric stop (**D**).

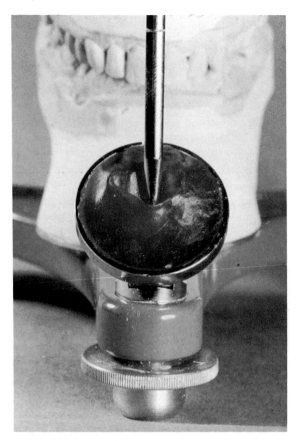

**Fig. 12.23** Customized incisal guidance table on the Dentatus ARH articulator.

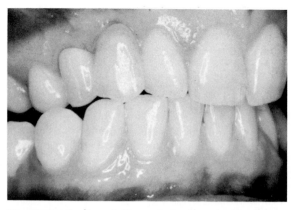

**Fig. 12.24** Cantilever bridge replacing 3| retained by 4| only. In lateral excursion, the occlusion is canine guided, and the pontic transmitted rotational forces to the premolar. The occlusal scheme should have been changed to group function to balance the forces on the bridge and the second premolar should have been included in the design.

functional pathways dictated by the teeth. When hard, the articulator will reproduce these movements when, say, a series of crowns is being constructed.

A change in the anterior guidance may be indicated when a key functional tooth is being replaced. This problem tends to be centred on the canine. If this tooth is lost in a canine guided occlusion, then consideration must be given to changing the occlusal scheme to group function, so that the prosthetic replacement, whether bridge pontic or denture tooth, is not subjected to unfavourable forces. Figure 12.24 shows a bridge replacing a canine, in lateral excursion. The pontic receives all the lateral load and transmits rotational forces to the premolar. This latter tooth was mobile and painful. The bridge required replacement and a change in the functional pattern to group function so that the lateral forces could be shared with other posterior teeth.

# 13. Extracoronal restorations

*G. J. Pearson*

The first phase in the treatment of the deep cavity was described in Chapter 10. In a posterior tooth, a large, and usually pinned, amalgam would be placed, and in an anterior tooth the result would be either a large composite resin restoration or more likely, because of dentine loss, the tooth would be committed to root canal therapy and a post crown.

The pinned amalgam might well give good service for some time, and it is certainly effective as a stabilization measure (Fig. 13.1). The large composite could do the same, pending root therapy. It may be, therefore, that these restorations would be used as the definitive treatment, or that further work could be planned to produce more functional and aesthetically pleasing restorations, usually meaning full crowns.

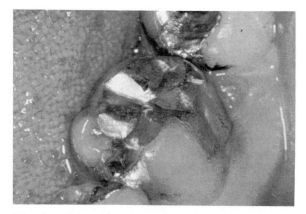

**Fig. 13.1** A large pinned amalgam, replacing one cusp, which would make a reasonable medium term restoration.

## TREATMENT PLANNING

The decision to crown depends not only on the individual tooth but on other general factors. These are:

- Patient motivation
- Oral hygiene status
- Periodontal condition
- The restorative state of the tooth
- Occlusal relationships

### Patient motivation

As was stressed in Section 1, patient motivation is essential, and any advanced operative work requires a commitment from both the patient and the dentist. The stabilization phase of the treatment plan will give the operator the opportunity to assess the patient's motivation, and, indeed, vice versa.

It is wise not to make any decision on the long term treatment until the patient's expectations and abilities have been assessed. Crowns must not be constructed just to placate a patient's vanity while other areas of the mouth are allowed to deteriorate. Crown preparation must be part of an agreed strategy aimed at the provision of a healthy mouth.

### Oral hygiene

Patients are frequently not made aware of their role in the maintenance of restorative dentistry and it is essential to instil this need to care from the start. The use of a plaque index will show the patient whether his attempts are effective and the simple illustration of the areas of plaque accumulation at each visit reinforces the educative process.

### Periodontal condition

Some years ago it was considered that crown placement on periodontally involved teeth was inappropriate. However, this attitude has changed

119

and now, once active periodontal disease has been controlled, it is frequently considered necessary to make extracoronal restorations to assist in the stabilization process. It is essential that the operator ensures that, in these circumstances, the restoration does not ruin all that the periodontist has achieved. Placement of margins, tooth reduction and crown contour are of critical importance in the production of a satisfactory result which will serve the patient for a reasonable period of time.

### Restorative state of the tooth

The checklist should ensure that the tooth is either vital or that adequate endodontic treatment has been carried out. An apical assessment with radiographs must be made. If there is doubt about the prognosis of a tooth, it is better not to embark on complex restorative work until the doubt has been removed. Nothing is more frustrating or embarrassing than to find the necessity for endodontics shortly after crown placement.

If the existing restoration had not been placed by the present operator and is of dubious quality, it should be removed. This is really part of the management of the deep cavity since the dentine can be examined to ensure it is caries free and the periphery may be examined to ensure that there is an adequate base of sound tooth upon which to place a crown margin. The remaining tooth can also be examined to decide on the techniques of core construction. An assessment of the tooth support likely to remain after crown preparation should be made so that weak undermined walls can be removed. This will influence the type and amount of additional retention to be provided for the core. It is usually best to plan for the worst and for the core to be well retained by an adequate number of pins.

The most common reason for crown construction is the fracture of one or more cusps. The position of the fracture line may well determine not only the type of restoration but also the fate of the tooth. Subgingival fractures are difficult to treat since the deeper they are, the more inaccessible they are to instruments and impression materials. Gingival surgery is often necessary to expose the margin and assess restorability.

### Occlusal relationships

The ability of an amalgam or composite resin to maintain occlusal stability will depend on the surface area of the restoration in contact with opposing supporting cusps and the accuracy with which the occlusal surface has been carved.

Once cusp or incisal tip loss has occurred, the prognosis for any direct restoration diminishes. While the restoration may not fail catastrophically, the effect of the oral environment on the physical properties of the material will result in slow degradation. The basis for this was discussed in Chapter 8; both amalgam and composite resin undergo creep, and the composite is vulnerable to surface deterioration. Occlusal loading leads to fatigue of both materials.

As a rule of thumb, one cusp can probably be restored reasonably with amalgam, but more than this and crowning should be considered. If an incisal edge is restored with composite resin then not only should the restoration itself be reviewed carefully, but also the opposing teeth, in case surface loss is caused by the hard filler particles of the composite (Fig. 13.2).

The tooth position relative to the adjacent and opposing teeth will influence the type of crown preparation to be used. Imbrication and rotation will alter the design of the preparation and may limit the ability to position its margins satisfactorily. Tilting of the adjacent teeth may limit the path of insertion of the restoration and prevent crown construction

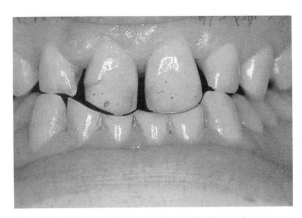

**Fig. 13.2** The extensive composite resin tips on the upper incisors, which have been present for some years, have abraded the lower incisors severely.

unless modifications are made to the approximal surfaces of these teeth as well.

The occlusal relationships should be studied prior to preparation. If there has been deterioration in these, then opposing cusps may be intruding beyond the planned occlusal plane and pre-operative equilibration of the area must be done (Ch. 12 and Fig. 12.19).

## PRINCIPLES OF PREPARATION

The preparation of any extracoronal restoration depends on planning the following:

- Path of insertion
- Stability of the restoration
- Margin position and type
- New occlusal relationships
- Choice of material

### Path of insertion

This is dictated by the approximal surfaces of the adjacent teeth and **not** by the long axis of the tooth to be prepared. Ignoring this may lead to an inability to seat the crown because its margin is obstructed by a tilted adjacent tooth.

The path of insertion is also linked to the stability of the restoration. A long, single path provides the maximum retention, and on tilted teeth, particularly lower molars, a lingually inclined path will provide the longest opposing walls.

### Stability of the restoration

This is the resistance provided by the preparation to displacing forces. These will usually be occlusal in origin and will give rise to rotational forces. Whilst retention is often considered in relation to the path of insertion, it is unlikely that displacing forces in service will act in this direction.

### Near-parallelism

Stability is achieved firstly by the principle of opposing parallel walls, which need to be based on the same level — parallel walls which are not on the same base do not provide stability (Fig. 13.3). The preparation of exactly parallel walls is difficult, and

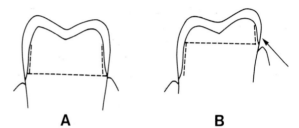

**Fig. 13.3** Stability in a full crown preparation. The parallel walls in preparation **A** are opposite each other on the same base, and provide excellent stability. The parallel walls in **B** are not on the same base, and the crown would be vulnerable to rotational forces.

near-parallelism, with an angle of convergence or taper of about five degrees is more realistic and achievable. Any increase in taper above this figure leads to a dramatic reduction in stability.

The tapered rotary instruments used in the preparation are manufactured with this taper, and so all that is required is to select the path of insertion and cut the entire periphery of the preparation with the bur held rigidly in this axis. The temptation to angle the bur for apparently easier access, particularly palatally, must be resisted, as this will produce far too much taper.

Basic retention will be created by a cervical collar resembling a squashed cylinder, which will occupy one-third to one-half of the crown height. The occlusal third of the buccal and lingual aspects will need to be curved, so that the overall reduction is even, and the final crown will not be bulbous (Fig. 13.4). Some teeth with short lingual walls will have less height bucco-lingually, and so attention must be paid to the approximal areas to create most of the retention.

Cutting the approximal surface can be made difficult by a long and broad contact area. Upper molars are a particular problem in that the contact is frequently wide and can extend down to the cervical margin.

### Crown height

A short clinical crown will increase the risk of failure by displacement since the path of insertion will be very short. Increasing the crown height may be achieved by gingival surgery, but this can produce very unsatisfactory results. Care must be taken to

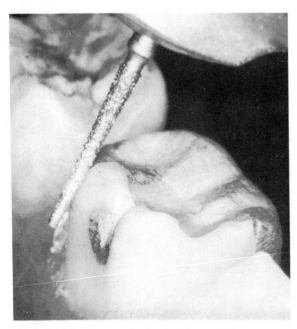

**Fig. 13.4** The bucco-occlusal reduction on a full veneer crown preparation. The cervical area provides the near-parallel collar for stability, and the remainder of the buccal wall must be reduced to conform with the contour of the tooth.

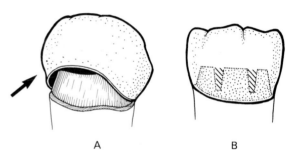

**Fig. 13.5** A short preparation (A) is vulnerable to lateral displacing forces. The incorporation of grooves (B) increases the resistance to displacement.

ensure that gross irregularities do not occur in the level of the gingival margin as a result of the lengthening of a single short wall.

Gingival surgery is probably of most use in the distal segment of the lower arch, where frequently the distal crown height of the last standing tooth is very short; the removal of a wedge of tissue can increase the crown height significantly.

The stability of short preparations can be increased by the use of slots and grooves. These will usually need to be placed in the buccal and lingual walls, though approximal grooves are useful where the lingual walls are short (Fig. 13.5).

If none of this is possible, then dentine pins incorporated in the casting will be the last resort.

### Occlusal reduction

Stability is increased by a preparation with a large surface area and having an occlusal surface which follows the proposed cusp outline. A flat topped preparation has less stability and also removes more tooth substance than is necessary.

### Margin position and type

The finishing margin of any crown is determined by the gingival contour, the restorative material to be used and the presence of any core.

Where aesthetics is not the primary consideration, the crown margin should be placed supragingivally to prevent plaque accumulation and subsequent gingival inflammation. The margin should therefore follow the sinuous outline of the gingival tissue, with no sharp changes of direction.

The margin should, however, extend beyond the junction of any core, so that it is sited on sound tooth. Failure to do this may lead to failure where the margin crosses the core/tooth junction, which will be vulnerable to recurrent caries.

The profile of the finishing line (Fig. 13.6) is determined by the material from which the crown will be constructed. Porcelain must have a *shoulder* with a minimum width of 1 mm, otherwise the material will be unsupported in thin section. Gold may be finished on a *chamfer* or a *bevelled shoulder*, the object being to achieve a 135° edge to the metal and to create a slip joint which can allow for slight casting shrinkage. This size of margin also allows the gold to be finished without running the risk of distortion.

The bevelled shoulder is used for partial veneer crowns where the supporting cusps require overlaying and the casting may be vulnerable to flexure. It may also be used for metal–ceramic crowns to provide margin strength for the subframe, and to provide a smoother enamel finish. The drawback to the bevelled shoulder is that it sacrifices a lot of tooth substance.

The chamfer is the principal finishing line for the veneer crown. It is conservative of tooth structure

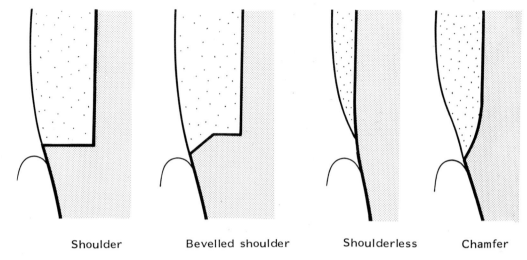

Shoulder     Bevelled shoulder     Shoulderless     Chamfer

**Fig. 13.6** Finishing line profiles for extracoronal restorations.

and provides clear definition of the extent of the preparation for both the clinician when reading the impression and the technician when waxing.

The *shoulderless* or knife-edge finishing line should not be used, as its definition is poor and can lead to inadequate thickness of metal, which may flex under load.

### New occlusal relationships

The new crown should harmonize with the existing occlusal relationships where they are satisfactory, but may be required to modify those that are not.

The occlusion should be examined pre-operatively for premature contacts and occlusal plane irregularities in the region of the proposed crown. If deterioration of the occlusal surface has occurred, the opposing tooth may have over-erupted. If this is not corrected, the new crown will continue the disharmony.

Crowns may also be used to correct rotations or aesthetic malalignments. The new crown position must be stable or the eventual result will be tooth movement and a worse problem subsequently (Figs 13.7, 13.8).

The occlusal clearance provided by the preparation must be sufficient to accommodate the chosen material (p. 112), and in load bearing areas there must be an adequate thickness to prevent

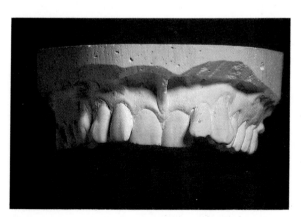

**Fig. 13.7** Pre-operative model showing proclined upper lateral incisors.

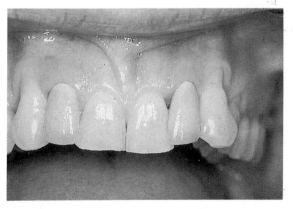

**Fig. 13.8** Porcelain jacket crowns re-aligning the lateral incisors. There is a danger in the class II division 2 case that the lip musculature will cause protrusion of the teeth again.

fracture. The shape of the reduction should indicate the cusp positions to the technician.

## Choice of material

The choice is between gold, ceramic and metal–ceramic. It is not intended to consider heat and light activated polymers since these are currently considered as provisional restoratives with limited life expectancy.

### Gold

Gold is still regarded as the most satisfactory extracoronal restorative material. It has a hardness similar to enamel, does not undergo creep intra-orally and may be cast accurately. The creation of the occlusal contour and axial surfaces is relatively straightforward by wax carving. It may be used in thin section and will allow the production of fine margins. It is not, however, regarded as a very aesthetic material.

There are a number of gold types with additions of other metals providing a variety of properties available for use in different parts of the mouth. The clinician should specify the type of gold required for each type of restoration (Table 13.1).

The reduction required to accommodate gold is approximately 1 mm throughout, and 1.5 mm, where possible, on the supporting cusps.

### Ceramic

Dental porcelain, or ceramic as it now termed, is regarded as the most aesthetic material used in the mouth, but is brittle and liable to fracture in thin section. It is essential to have a minimum thickness of 0.8 mm at the margin and at least 1–1.5 mm incisally. It is not strong enough to be used alone for full crowns on posterior teeth or for bridgework. Its weakness is that cracks can originate from micropores on the fit surface, and that these can open catastrophically in tension or bending. They resist compression well. Therefore the principle of the preparation is to provide dentine support for the ceramic throughout, particularly on the incisal and cingulum areas.

Dental porcelain is harder than enamel and the **unglazed** surface will abrade tooth surface and frequently results in considerable wear to the opposing tooth (Fig. 13.9).

### Metal–ceramic

The bonding of metal and ceramic has revolutionized practice in crown and bridgework. The combination provides good aesthetics and excellent strength. Its disadvantage is that it requires considerable tooth reduction to accommodate it. This particularly applies to the occlusal aspect where 2 mm clearance is desirable if ceramic is to cover the occlusal surface. Other areas for which ceramic coverage is desired

**Table 13.1** Properties of cast gold types I–IV gold alloys

|  | Type I | Type II | Type III | Type IV |
|---|---|---|---|---|
| Composition |  |  |  |  |
| Au (%) | 81–83 | 76–78 | 73–77 | 71–74 |
| Pt(%) | – | – | – | 0.1 |
| Pl(%) | 0.2–4.5 | 1.3 | 2.4 | 2.5 |
| Fusion temperature (°C) | 930 | 900 | 900 | 870 |
| Tensile strength (MN/mm) | 285–315 | 315–420 | 510–550 | 750–900 |
| Yield strength (MN/mm) | 100–110 | 150–185 | 290–310 | 480–510 |
| Hardness | 60–70 | 95–140 | 150–170 | 220–250 |
| Use | Inlays in very low stress areas | All types of simple inlay | Crowns, ¾ crowns, cuspal coverage inlays | Partial dentures |

All mechanical properties are measured with the alloys in their hardened state.

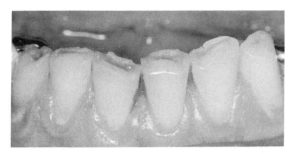

**Fig. 13.9** Lower incisors which have been in contact with poorly glazed porcelain for some years. There is considerable surface loss.

should have a 1.5 mm reduction, which should be evenly removed from the whole surface contour. This means that the final third of the preparation will curve markedly towards the occlusal aspect. This is frequently the main fault during preparation. Two problems follow from this:

1. The technician overbuilds the crown to give adequate thickness of material for aesthetics. The crown is then grossly overbuilt (Fig. 13.10A);
2. The technician attempts to maintain the original tooth anatomy which leads to a thinning of the ceramic and metal, with poor aesthetics and the subsequent fracture of the porcelain occlusally (Fig. 13. 10B).

The choice of material for the functional surfaces must also be considered. Glazed porcelain is usually the patient's choice but it is difficult to produce the anatomical form accurately and adjust it intra-orally. If not reglazed, it will damage the opposing tooth surface. Metal is therefore preferred.

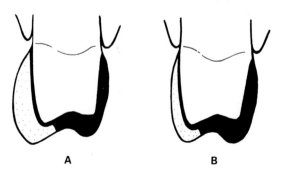

**Fig. 13.10** Incorrect preparation for metal–ceramic crowns and the consequences. **A**, The crown is made bulbous to reproduce the correct shade; **B**, The correct contour is reproduced, but this means that the ceramic is too thin.

# DEVELOPMENTS IN MATERIALS

## Ceramics

The major development in dental ceramics alone was the introduction of fine crystals of fused alumina into a glass of matched thermal expansion, with consequent dispersion strengthening of the ceramic. The aluminous crown was introduced in the mid-1960s, and the improvement of physical properties achieved by this has not really been surpassed.

Some other suggestions, such as ion strengthening, require long immersion or complex treatments, which are not suited to commercial laboratories.

The introduction of a tin oxide coated, bonded platinum foil, the twin foil technique, has the claimed advantage of helping the ceramic resist the static fatigue which occurs as a result of water immersion. However, the clinical and laboratory results of studies on this system are so contradictory that its value remains unproven.

### Castable ceramic

More recently, castable ceramics have become available. The crowns are produced by the lost wax technique, as used in the preparation of gold restorations. This ensures that the occlusal morphology is accurate and requires little modification. The other advantage of these materials is that the risk of abrasion is reduced since the material has a similar hardness value to enamel. Colouring is applied to the outer surface of the crown and the durability of this system is as yet uncertain.

## Bonding alloys

The most reliable and successful method for strengthening ceramics is the provision of a cast metal subframe, which prevents the propagation of cracks from the ceramic inner surface. Developments in the alloys for this purpose have been rapid, and the materials available are discussed in Chapter 18.

# RESTORATION OF ROOT FILLED TEETH

By the time caries and/or trauma has destroyed coronal dentine and the endodontic access cavity has been cut, there will usually be little dentine remaining to support a crown. Should a crown therefore be required on a root filled tooth, some form of core will need to be constructed to retain it and provide stability.

The post crown, where the core is itself retained by a post in the root canal, has some limitations. These relate to the morphology and size of the roots.

Where the root is very variable and cannot be seen clearly by radiography, the post crown is a real hazard (Ch. 21). This is true of posterior teeth, particularly those which are sometimes one- and sometimes two-rooted. The two-rooted premolar may also have very narrow roots, quite unsuitable for receiving posts.

In these circumstances, it is safer to provide a pin retained amalgam core, rather than embark on a split cast device. If there is not enough dentine for the pins, then the root canals can be used for retention, but using small cemented preformed posts which only intrude by about 3 mm into the canal.

In the anterior teeth, the post and core is the restoration of choice.

## Posts and cores

There is a huge range of post and core systems from which to choose.

They may be classified into:

- Cast
- Prefabricated
- Hybrid

### Cast post and core

Here the natural shape of the canal is used, after the elimination of undercuts and irregularities, to form a conical preparation. The post shape may be recorded either by using the direct technique with inlay wax or a non-residual burnout acrylic, or indirectly by taking an elastomeric impression. The core is waxed to the appropriate shape for the particular tooth and the system has the major advantage that it is made to fit the tooth, rather than the tooth being prepared to fit the system.

The major disadvantage of the cast post is that it is weaker than the equivalent diameter of a wrought post. Therefore, if fracture of the post is to be avoided, the diameter of the canal must be enlarged to ensure

an adequate bulk of metal. This means that the technique sacrifices more tooth and weakens the root in comparison with the prefabricated systems.

The cast post is probably the technique of choice for large canals, for difficult alignment problems, and when a cast diaphragm is required to support the root, or make up subgingival deficiencies.

### Prefabricated post and core

These posts are factory-made in a range of sizes with a matching twist drill system to prepare the root canal to receive the post.

The posts may be *parallel sided* or *tapered* and these in turn may be *smooth, serrated, threaded* or *vented*. The choice is immense and personal preference has a large part to play in selection. Of the various types, the tapered threaded post is the most dangerous, since its insertion can generate enough stress to split the root.

The majority of non-threaded posts are made of stainless steel and are therefore strong in narrow diameters, whilst the threaded systems tend to be brass.

Parallel posts are effective in most teeth, but care must be taken with them in small roots, because the danger of perforation of the canal wall is high. Tapered posts are better in narrow canals.

The vented posts allow room for the escape of excess cement and are therefore claimed to permit better seating.

Perhaps the biggest drawback of the basic system is that the core position, size and shape is relatively fixed. Some modifications are possible, but are limited in extent. The biggest claimed advantage is that they remove one laboratory stage, and are therefore more economical.

### Hybrid — post prefabricated, cast core

This group has prefabricated posts with a custom made core cast onto the post. This combines the strength of the wrought post which is either semi-precious alloy or nickel–chromium, with the advantage of being able to shape the core exactly for the particular tooth.

Figure 13.11 shows the Wiptam technique which utilizes a smooth parallel-sided nickel–cobalt–chromium wire, which fits into a matched preparation. The core is cast gold, and extends into a

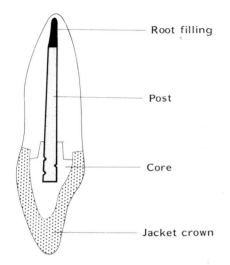

**Fig. 13.11** The Wiptam post crown.

countersink to reinforce the post and provide resistance to rotation. The shoulder, which receives the crown is cut separately, which may leave a collar of dentine that effectively lengthens the canal preparation. The collar must have sufficient bulk so that it does not fracture on the die. Some systems provide plastic burnout posts which can be used instead of the metal ones, but these create some problems.

The narrower posts are flexible and will negotiate curves which the final post will not, and the disadvantages of the cast post mentioned above are reintroduced.

The core waxing may be done either in the mouth or in the laboratory.

### Canal preparation

Whatever system is used, there are a number of common features in the preparations. The following aspects are important:

- Root canal morphology
- Length
- Diameter
- Rotation resistance
- Core characteristics

***Root canal morphology.*** Assessment of the root canal morphology is required before committing the tooth to a post preparation. It is essential to have an adequate apical seal and the root filling material should be removable from the coronal end of the canal. A full length silver point is a considerable nuisance, and should be replaced with gutta percha if possible. If it cannot be removed, then a post will be impossible, and a pinned core will have to be considered.

The cross-section of the canal and the presence of any curvature should be assessed. A very narrow canal may make preparation difficult and an excessive curvature may limit the extent of the post and reduce retention. It should also be remembered that the radiograph only shows curves mesially or distally, and not labially or palatally.

***Length.*** The length of the post is one of the most critical features. A short post is capable of exerting enough leverage to split the root when loaded transversely. It also determines in part its retention and the longer the post, the greater the load bearing area for dissipation of forces to the surrounding bone. As a rule of thumb, the post should be as long as the crown it is expected to retain.

***Diameter.*** The diameter is determined by the anatomy of the canal, the amount of diseased tooth tissue removed and the type of metal used in the post and core construction. In order not to weaken the root, the post should not be more than one-third the total root width for the whole root length. This suggests superiority for the tapered post.

However, if the parallel post obeys the rule in the apical danger zone, it will be narrower coronally. This is how the addition of the custom core adapts the parallel post to fulfil ideal requirements, since the diameter is increased by the cast-on metal. The prefabricated core type does not do this, except on the Schenker type (Fig. 13.12).

The range of post diameters which are successful is 1.2–1.5 mm.

***Rotation resistance.*** A cylindrical post will rotate under stress from the occlusion and may not locate accurately when tried in. Some prefabricated systems require the cutting of grooves or notches to provide resistance to rotation.

However, the natural shape of the root canal is oval and it seems a pity not to utilize this natural feature and to avoid the stress concentrations and weakness created by antirotational notches.

The canal can be simply enlarged coronally to follow the root contour smoothly and this area can be engaged by cast-on core.

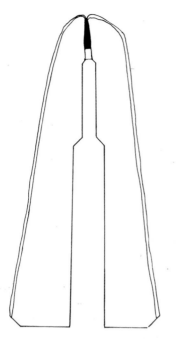

**Fig. 13.12** The Schenker post. It is parallel sided, but is stepped down to reduce the apical diameter.

***Core characteristics.*** The core should provide retention and stability for the final restoration and should be similar to the shape of a conventional crown preparation (Fig. 13.13).

It is possible to realign the position of the crown with the core, which allows derotation or uprighting relative to the root position. However, this option must be used with caution since there is frequently an interplay between the hard and soft tissues, and muscle pressure may well move the altered tooth producing a bizarre result.

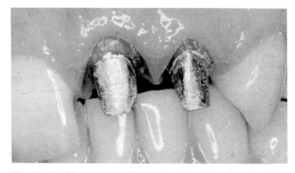

**Fig. 13.13** Two posts and cores in place, showing that the basic core shape is similar to the porcelain jacket crown preparation, but is smaller.

The core can also be smaller than the vital tooth preparation since there is no pulp to worry about. This gives added bulk to the final crown, which is a considerable advantage for the strength of a porcelain crown, and helps the aesthetics of the metal–ceramic crown.

## PROVISIONAL CROWNS

This aspect of advanced operative work is frequently neglected and little time is devoted to the construction of a good provisional crown.

The functions of a provisional crown are:

- Protection of cut dentine
- Maintenance of the occlusion
- Maintenance of approximal contacts
- Restoration of aesthetics
- Maintenance of gingival health

It is good practice to construct the provisional crown prior to the impression of the preparation, since this will allow proper estimation of the time remaining for this.

Provisional crowns may be customized or made from prefabricated crown forms.

### Customized crowns

An impression in putty is taken prior to the start of the preparation and put to one side. On completion of the preparation the putty impression is used to form a mould for a resin based material. This sets to the shape of the original crown. Once polymerization has completed, the impression and crown are removed and the resin trimmed accurately to the margins of the preparation and the occlusion, and polished. The provisional should be cemented with a weak ZOE cement.

### Prefabricated crowns

Anterior crown forms can be tooth coloured, usually polycarbonate or transparent cellulose acetate. They are available in a range of sizes for each tooth and the size should be chosen to conform to the mesio-distal width. They need to be cut carefully to the cervical margins and then based with a self-curing resin (Fig. 13.14).

The range of sizes can be restrictive; it can be

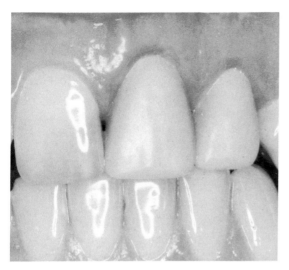

**Fig. 13.14** Provisional restorations for the case shown in Fig. 13.13. They have been made from transparent crown forms, and provide correct aesthetics, occlusion and gingival contour.

difficult to find one with the correct dimensions both bucco-lingually and mesio-distally.

Posteriorly, the best provisional crowns are anatomically shaped silver–tin crowns. These are also designed as burnout patterns for crown waxing. They are soft and can be adapted easily to the occlusion and to the cervical margin. They do not usually require basing with a resin, and can be cemented with a stiff ZOE cement. Their disadvantage is that being soft, they have a limited life.

## IMPRESSIONS AND SHADE

These are discussed in Chapters 17 and 18.

## CEMENTATION

The sequence for cementation is:

1. Check the restoration on the model before the patient arrives, ensuring that there are contacts with adjacent teeth and that the occlusion is correct. Examine the die and the adjacent teeth on the model for rub marks which may have introduced errors;

2. Do not attempt cementation if the tooth displays any adverse symptoms. If the patient complains of discomfort, diagnose the cause and treat it before cementation;

3. Remove the provisional and clean the preparation, ensuring that all cement is removed. If possible this should be done without local analgesic since this can prevent the patient assisting in the assessment of the occlusion;

4. Try in the restoration. If it does not seat initially check the contacts with floss. If the restoration still does not seat, the fit surface should be examined and if necessary a silcone rubber perfecting paste may be used to detect any high spots;

5. Once the crown has been seated, check the marginal adaptation. There should be a smooth transition from the tooth onto the crown. Check the shade in daylight;

6. The occlusal contacts should be assessed. Premature contacts may be detected using either articulating paper or shimstock. The type of articulating paper can affect the results since some are excessively thick and will not allow for differentiation of the high points and normal occlusal stops. Fine articulating paper is preferable and it is often advantageous for the occlusal surface of the restoration to have a matt finish in order to detect the minor prematurities which may be present.

The occlusal contacts must be checked in all excursions. Heavy contacts must be eased but care should be taken that the surface is not over-reduced, since this will take the crown out of occlusion;

7. *Choice of cement.* Incorrect selection and manipulation of the cement will affect the life of a crown dramatically.

The main luting agents are also bases and these were discussed in Chapter 9. There are two choices for cementation. One provides mechanical retention (ZOE or zinc phosphate) and the other provides this, and adhesion to tooth and some adhesion to the restoration. Clearly, the second is preferable and zinc polycarboxylate and glass ionomer cements have become popular. The polycarboxylate is the more reliable since there is some concern about the pulpal response to glass ionomers when used as luting materials.

The cement should be mixed to the manufacturer's specified powder/liquid ratio which should provide a consistency that will allow it to be displaced as the crown is seated and excess will flow away;

8. The fit surface of the crown should be coated

with cement, placed on the preparation, which has been isolated and dried, and seated home. Considerable pressure should be applied to the seating crown initally to express the excess cement and

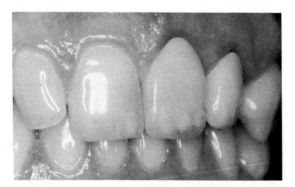

**Fig. 13.15** The finished crowns. These show the characterization that the skilled ceramist can produce. Note the translucency at the tips and the incorporation of white flecks.

pressure should be maintained until the cement has set. For a post crown, the canal should be cleaned, and filled with cement prior to seating the post and crown together with the same mix;

9. Once the cement has set, excess is fractured away from the margin and the approximal embrasures cleared with floss.

10. After cementation, the occlusal relationship should be rechecked (Fig. 13.15).

## REVIEW

The crown should be inspected again a week or so later, since natural occlusal function will have been re-established, and contacts may require further adjustment.

Radiographic review should be carried out six months later and every two years or so, to check for silent development of apical pathology.

# 14. Adhesive techniques

## G. J. Pearson

True adhesive dentistry stemmed from the invention by Michael Bounocore in 1955 of the acid etch technique, but it took Ray Bowen's development of bis-GMA resin to make further progress. Since the late 1960s, many techniques have evolved using essentially these two inventions as their basis.

Buonocore demonstrated that the application of phosphoric acid to enamel would cause preferential dissolution of the interprismatic substance. This resulted in a roughened surface with a series of micropores into which a fluid resin would flow.

*Enamel bonding agents* are mainly unfilled, diluted bis-GMA resins which can be used alone as fissure sealants, or coupled with composite resin. They have good wetting properties and their penetration of the micropores forms *tags* of up to 50 $\mu$m long. After polymerization, the tags interlock solidly with the enamel to provide excellent mechanical union. This union provides retention and good resistance to microleakage.

The applications of the technique have progressed from fissure sealing and class IV restorations, through composite and resin veneers, to resin retained bridges and ceramic veneers. Together with dentine bonding agents, the technique is also used for the improvement of the marginal adaptation and stability of intracoronal restorations (Ch. 9).

## VENEERS

### Composite resin veneers

In cases of hypoplastic defects of enamel, intrinsic staining and mild malformations, the acid etch technique was used without tooth reduction to bond a layer of composite resin to the tooth to mask or reshape the defect.

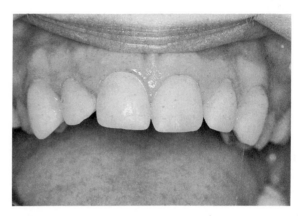

**Fig. 14.1** Composite resin veneers on 321|123.

The absence of tooth reduction led to bulbous labial contours and attendant gingival problems. The technique progressed by the use of a half enamel thickness reduction to accommodate the resin, and the development of opaquing resins and an increased number of shades of translucent resins. Variations and gradations of shade could be incorporated (Fig. 14.1).

However, composite resins tend to stain and lose their surface, and so the veneers were semi-permanent, and could require replacement every two years or so.

### Polycarbonate resin veneers

In parallel with the composite resin veneers came the development of factory-made polycarbonate resin veneers. Again, originally no tooth reduction was recommended, with the appropriately sized veneer being bonded in place by a large amount of composite (Fig. 14.2).

Tooth reduction, accompanied by a laboratory

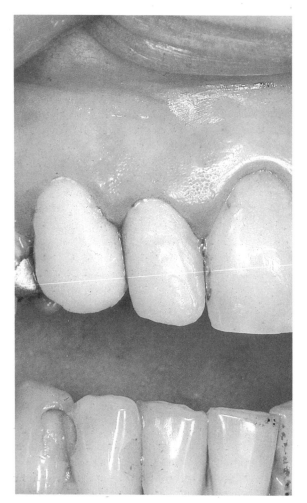

**Fig. 14.2** Polycarbonate resin facings on 32|. They are bulbous because no labial reduction has been done.

stage to shape the veneer more accurately, made this technique more acceptable, but it has been largely superseded by the ceramic veneer.

### Ceramic veneers

These utilize the half-enamel thickness reduction and the acid etch technique to bond a thin layer of ceramic to the tooth.

They are a valuable alternative to the porcelain jacket crown for correction of unsightly enamel defects, and originated in the 1920s when Pincus made veneers which fell off because they were poorly attached to the enamel.

The bonding agents in current use are those which are used to cement resin retained bridges (p. 137), together with composite resins which can be used to mask strong underlying colours or modify the shade of the veneer. The mode of adhesion to the ceramic relies on etching or sand blasting and then coating the fit surface with a silane coupling agent (Ch.18).

Adhesion is much better to enamel than to dentine and the best results are obtained with either complete attachment to enamel or, where enamel has been lost, with at least 1 mm of enamel present around the periphery of the restoration. If too much dentine is present, then crowns are a better alternative.

The preparation (Fig. 14.3) involves the reduction of a half-enamel thickness over the whole surface, which means that there is a variable thickness of enamel removal. The reduction is extended into the approximal embrasures and should, if at all possible, remain on enamel.

Defects, such as acid erosion, should be made good with glass ionomer cement and some operators even suggest that the erosion lesion should be deepened to allow a minimum thickness of 0.5 mm of glass ionomer cement to be placed. The finishing margin should be a narrow shoulder or chamfer to support the delicate ceramic structure.

Several preparation designs have been suggested depending upon the need to cover the incisal edge.

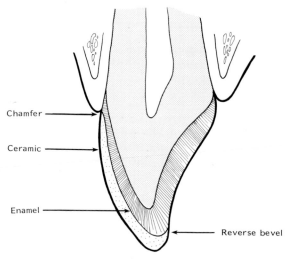

**Fig. 14.3** Diagram of the preparation for a ceramic veneer. It removes half the enamel thickness, has a supra-gingival cervical finishing line, and an incisal reverse bevel to increase the thickness of ceramic on the incisal edge.

4. Prime the metal, if required;
5. Place the cement on the bridge and seat home;
6. Remove excess prior to setting and place oxygen barrier;
7. Adjust the occlusion.

The treatment of a typical case is shown in Figure 14.10.

### Selection of cement

There are three types of cement:

- Conventional restorative composites
- Conventional resin luting cements
- Dual affinity resins

Most cements are chemically cured although a number of 'dual cure' materials are available which are initiated by visible light but also contain a chemical initiator. This means that polymerization will take place even when the light does not reach the full thickness of the material.

The conventional resins rely on mechanical retention and because of the high filler loading, they are only suitable for use in large mesh bridges.

The conventional luting cements are dilute forms of the restorative resins with less filler of smaller particle size. They often contain lower molecular weight resins as diluents. Again retention to enamel and metalwork is mechanical.

Newer single and dual affinity resins will bond chemically to tooth structure and to the metalwork. These are based on 4-methacryloxyethyl trimellitic acid anhydride (4-meta), 4-meta with methyl methacrylate, 4-meta with bis-GMA or the halogenated phosphate ester of bis-GMA. Some of these have shown very high bond strengths to enamel, and apparently offer advantages over the purely mechanical retention given by the other types of cement.

### Debonding

This presents the main problem and will occur either almost immediately after placement, or will be delayed some time.

In the first instance the debond is associated with contamination during cementation and failure of the tooth adhesive interface. Later failures can occur at either of the two interfaces but, increasingly, evidence of failure within the cements has been found. Debonding appears to be more common in cases where multiple abutments have been used.

When partial debonding occurs, it is essential that the bridge is removed and re-cemented, otherwise there is a high risk of recurrent caries under the loose wing.

If the bond to the other abutment is too good, removal will be very difficult. Here, a window can be cut in the loose wing, and it can be converted to the old Rochette design. The tooth can be re-etched through the window and composite placed afterwards to resecure the wing. Alternatively, the loose wing can be cut off and the bridge thereby converted to a cantilever type.

## CONCLUSION

This is a rapidly developing field, both in the area of adhesive materials and in the accumulation of clinical experience. It will be some years before definitive judgements and recommendations can be made on the clinical indications and techniques for adhesive dentistry.

# 15. Bridgework — treatment planning and design

## P. H. Jacobsen

## DEFINITIONS

A bridge is a false tooth, or teeth, permanently attached to natural teeth. The false tooth, the *pontic*, is joined by *connectors* to *retainers*, which may be either inlays or crowns, which in turn are cemented to *abutment teeth* (Fig. 15.1).

The pontic may be *fixed* rigidly to the retainer, or it may have a *movable* joint. Bridges may be classified according to the type of connectors either side of the pontic, as either *fixed–fixed* or *fixed–movable*. In addition, the pontic may only have one connector and be free at the other end — this is a *cantilever bridge*. If the pontic is some distance away from the retainer, and the connector is a metal bar, this is a *spring cantilever bridge*.

Bridges are also referred to by the total number of retainers and pontics; for example, a *five unit* bridge.

## DESIGN CONSIDERATIONS

### Biological factors

The longevity of bridgework depends firstly on the biological integrity and prognosis of each abutment

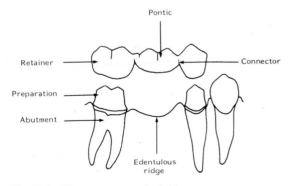

**Fig. 15.1** The components of a bridge.

tooth. The crown must be caries free and the pulp must either be healthy, or be replaced by a sound root filling with no apical pathology. The periodontium must also be healthy and well maintained. Teeth that have suffered previous periodontal breakdown are not excluded from being abutments, but the disease must have been stabilized and the plaque control maintained at a high level.

The number of abutments required to support the proposed pontics is often a matter of opinion. Ante proposed that the combined root surface area of the abutment teeth should be equal or greater than that of the teeth to be replaced. This seems to assume that the abutments will be subjected to greater loading, possibly up to one and a half times more.

However, work from Scandinavia, where extensive bridges were provided for periodontally dubious teeth, together with clinical experience, suggests that Ante's law is over-cautious, and that occlusal loading is modified by a bio-feedback mechanism to a level appropriate to the support available.

Rather than looking at the axial occlusal loads on abutments, it seems more important to consider the possible leverage and torque that may be applied. This will arise during function and para-function in lateral excursions, and the assessment of the occlusion is crucial in bridge design. For example, in a canine guided occlusion, lateral stresses on posterior teeth are small, and perhaps this is more favourable for abutments.

This is not to say that a large number of pontics can be supported by a few abutments, because retention of the bridge is also important, rather that bridges made with less than the traditionally ideal level of support, can be clinically successful.

The root surface area of the abutment teeth is clearly important, though, with the upper canine and the upper first molar having the largest areas, which make them ideal for bridge support, whilst at the other end of the scale, the upper lateral incisor has a very small root, and is often unsuitable as a terminal abutment. Pragmatically, then, it would seem sensible to adopt designs that utilize the teeth with the largest root surface areas available in the particular circumstances.

## Mechanical factors

Each abutment tooth must also be mechanically sound. It must either have dentine of sufficient quality and quantity to allow the preparation of a retentive crown, or it must be capable of being restored, depending upon its position, by a pinned core or a post and core.

The abutment preparations for a fixed–fixed bridge must be parallel. The bridge will eventually be inserted in one piece and this will not be possible if each preparation has a different path of insertion.

Each preparation should provide excellent mechanical retention, achieved by near parallism of walls (Ch.13) and, it used to be said, that in a fixed–fixed bridge, the retention of each retainer should be approximately the same. This rule would preclude the use of a premolar and molar retaining a pontic between them, without the use of a non-rigid connector. However, clinical experience suggests that provided each tooth has **good** retention, such a bridge would be successful.

Previously, a movable joint would be used as a stress breaker, balancing the loads transmitted to each tooth, but this concept is currently out of fashion, with the vast majority of connectors being rigid soldered joints. However, there are other indications for the non-rigid connector.

First, it may be used where an intracoronal inlay retains one end of a bridge, whilst the other is retained by an occlusal coverage restoration. Loads applied to the inlayed tooth only, could displace this independently of the bridge, thus stressing its cement lute. If the connector to this *minor retainer* was non-rigid, then some small independent movement would be allowed. However, because of the development of the resin-retained bridge, intracoronal inlays are rarely indicated as bridge retainers.

Secondly, and more importantly, a movable joint can solve the problems of non-parallel alignment of

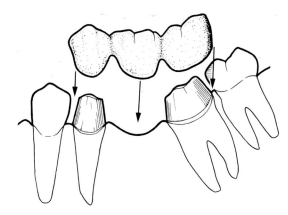

**Fig. 15.2**  Tilted teeth — the problem of a fixed–fixed bridge. The seating of the bridge is prevented by the mesial aspect of the last molar, even though the preparations have been cut with a common path of insertion.

abutment teeth. Whilst a common path of insertion could be cut for both retainers shown in Figure 15.2, a fixed–fixed bridge would be prevented from seating by the mesial aspect of the last molar.

The malaligned tooth, or teeth, could possibly be uprighted orthodontically, but this may not always be practical. To overcome this, the path of insertion of the retainer on the tilted abutment can be made in the long axis of that tooth, and a movable joint made in the crown on the minor retainer, parallel to the path of insertion of the bridge (Fig 15.3). The dovetail slot may either be milled in the casting, or be a preformed precision retainer (Fig 15.4). An alternative way of overcoming discrepancies in paths of insertion, is to use telescopic crowns (Fig 15.5).

## Aesthetic factors

This may well be one of the major reasons for providing bridgework and a decision must be made about which teeth should have tooth coloured components had which can remain all metal. The all-metal retainer utilizes a minimal preparation and is technically less demanding than an aesthetic one.

The aesthetic component has to have space in the preparation to accommodate it and requires higher technical skills for its construction, particularly if it is to function in the occlusion.

Facing materials tend to be applied directly to a metal sub-frame, and may be ceramics or resin-based composites. The use of pre-formed cemented facings,

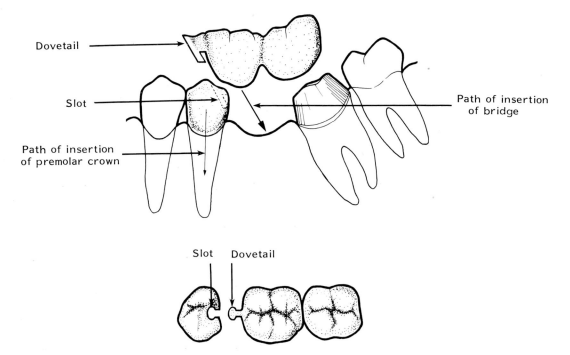

**Fig. 15.3**   Tilted teeth — the fixed-movable bridge. Each abutment has a preparation cut in its long axis. The crown on the premolar has a dovetail shaped slot cut in its distal aspect (the preparation must be reduced to accommodate it) and the pontic has the dovetail shaped piece to fit the slot. The line of the dovetail is the path of insertion of the molar preparation.

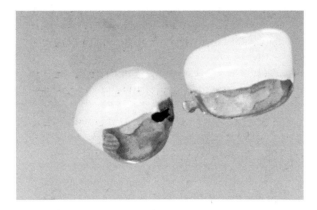

**Fig. 15.4**   A precision retainer, e.g. the Sterngold Tubelock, can be used as a movable joint.

such as Steele's long pin type, has largely died out.

Wherever possible, and with the agreement of the patient, the occlusal surfaces should be reproduced in metal (Ch. 12).

If the purpose of the bridge is to alter the aesthetics, then this must be carefully planned at the diagnostic stage (p. 144).

## Retainers

The choice is essentially between intracoronal inlays, partial veneer crowns or full crowns. For simplicity of preparation and reliability of fit, the full crown has become the most used, though sometimes overused retainer. The overprescription of ceramic fused to metal is partly responsible for this.

However, the preparation of complex intracoronal shapes or long external margins makes the retainer more demanding for both the clinician and the technician, so inlays and partial veneer crowns should be reserved for those special occasions, which in practical terms are very few.

The clear advantage of the partial veneer is that it leaves the buccal surface of the tooth intact. This can be aesthetically pleasing and conservative of tooth tissue.

## Pontics

These will always have a functional component, and will often have an aesthetic one as well.

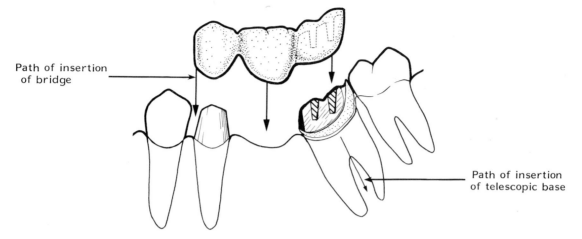

Path of insertion
of bridge

Path of insertion
of telescopic base

**Fig. 15.5** Tilted teeth — the telescopic crown. The preparations are in the long axis of each tooth. A gold coping is made for the molar, which is milled to receive a partial veneer crown with slots and grooves. The path of insertion of the bridge is then aligned with the premolar preparation.

For its functional aspects, the pontic should provide occlusal stability by inclusion of centric stops and supporting cusps as appropriate. Its participation in the new occlusal scheme should be decided (p. 116) and it should not create any interferences.

All the above could be fulfilled by a flat plate of metal and the *wash-through* or *sanitary* pontics (Fig. 15.6) are useful from the periodontal viewpoint, in that the tissues around the pontic can be readily cleaned. However, their use is usually confined to the molar region, and is rare because of their aesthetic limitations.

The majority of pontics will need to be aesthetic and this will mean the inclusion of a tooth coloured facing in conjunction with the metal functional surface.

The aesthetic component will need to reproduce the embrasure spaces and contact the soft tissue of the alveolar ridge. This contact must be firm, but not intrusive to reduce plaque accumulation under the pontic.

The tissue contact should be confined to the buccal or labial aspect of the ridge, with the remainder accessible to the tongue (Fig. 15.7).

If tissue loss has been extensive, pink porcelain may be necessary at the neck of the pontic, or alternatively, a removable pontic with gumwork should be considered (p. 150).

**Fig. 15.6** A sanitary pontic, retained by two partial veneer crowns.

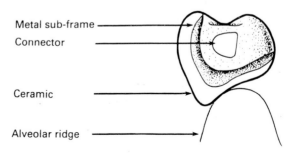

Metal sub-frame

Connector

Ceramic

Alveolar ridge

**Fig. 15.7** The ridge contact of a premolar pontic.

Special oral hygiene techniques are required to maintain the undersurface of the pontics and connectors in a plaque free condition, and the most useful aid is Superfloss (Fig. 15.8).

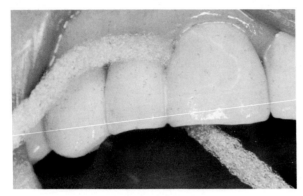

**Fig. 15.8**  Superfloss being used to clean the embrasures and fitting surface of an anterior pontic.

## INDICATIONS FOR BRIDGEWORK

Not every missing tooth needs to replaced, and where several teeth are missing, a partial denture may be a more sensible option.

For instance, it is not necessary to replace a missing molar whose loss has not detracted from occlusal stability. Inter- and intra-arch relationships can be monitored, and a replacement advised if there is evidence of deterioration.

Aesthetics tends to be a major motivating factor for the patient, as is the desire to replace an existing partial denture.

### Bridge versus partial denture

All partial dentures are potentially harmful and it can be argued that a bridge is very desirable to avoid the presence of a denture base, connectors and clasps. However, it is clear that not every mouth with missing teeth should be restored with bridgework and the following should be borne in mind:

- The number and position of missing teeth
- The periodontal condition of abutment teeth
- Angulation of abutment teeth
- Plaque and caries control
- Patient motivation and other general factors (Ch. 4)
- Clinical and technical skills available
- Economic factors

The larger the number of missing teeth and the poorer the periodontal support of the remainder, the more the partial denture is the sensible option. However, plaque control must be good for both options and active caries must be controlled.

Extensive bridgework is beyond the training of many general dental practitioners and their technicians, and it is much wiser to admit this than to embark on restorations that could fail. Remember, a failed bridge is potentially more hazardous than a failed partial denture (Ch. 21).

Finally, the patient will have to pay for the bridge and maintain it when it is inserted. Without the assurance that the patient can keep the bridge in a plaque and caries free condition, the restoration should not be attempted.

### Conventional bridgework versus resin-retained bridgework

The upsurge in the use of adhesive bridgework of various designs, and its long term success, has meant considerable reduction in the indications for bridgework retained by inlays and crowns. Certainly, short spans with moderately sound abutment teeth are best treated by adhesive bridgework. But in a rapidly developing area, it is difficult to provide definitive indications in other circumstances. Long spans in the posterior regions and lower incisor regions can be successful, but upper anterior teeth present the problems of unfavourable displacing forces (Table 15.1).

The more heavily restored the potential abutment

**Table 15.1**  Indications and advantages for resin retained bridgework

| Indications | Contraindications | Advantages | Disadvantages |
|---|---|---|---|
| Short spans | Long spans | Technically simple | Metal visible through tooth |
| Sound enamel available | Heavily restored teeth | Cheap | Debonding problems |
| Favourable occlusion | Multiple upper anterior teeth | | |

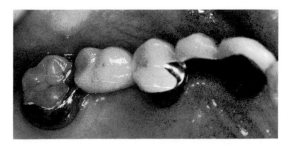

**Fig. 15.9**   The hybrid resin retained bridge. This five unit fixed–fixed bridge has been retained by full crowns on the canine and second premolar, and by a resin retained wing on the second molar. The natural occlusion and considerable tooth tissue has been maintained on the molar.

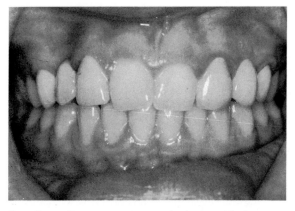

**Fig. 15.10**   The upper canines are in the lateral incisor positions, and two bridges have been made to replace the lost deciduous canines. There is incorrect disproportion between the sizes of the new laterals, canines, and the original central incisors because the canines cannot be reduced enough to resemble incisors.

tooth is, the more likely it is that there will not be enough enamel remaining for bonding — crowns are a better option. The hybrid design also has potential: one abutment could have a conventional crown, whilst another, with more enamel, could have a resin-retained wing (Fig. 15.9).

In sound mouths, the resin-retained bridge is now the treatment of choice for short spans, with conventional bridges reserved for more extensive cases.

## PRE-OPERATIVE CONSIDERATIONS FOR CONVENTIONAL BRIDGEWORK

### The patient

The patient must be well motivated, clearly informed of his responsibilities in maintaining the proposed restoration and understand the sequence of appointments and what is to be achieved at each. He must be capable of maintaining good plaque control and any caries, periodontal disease and poor restorations must have been stabilized.

### The occlusion

A pre-operative precentric mounting and analysis should have been performed (Ch. 12) and consideration given to possible tooth movement in order to achieve more favourable tooth relationships.

Orthodontics has a crucial role to play in mouth preparation where there are malposed teeth or uneven spacing, particularly anteriorly. For example, conversion of a canine to a lateral incisor as part of a bridge restoring the space left by a retained deciduous canine can be very difficult (Fig. 15.10). It

is often more desirable to move teeth into their correct positions first and in the case illustrated, a better aesthetic result would have been achieved if the canine had been moved distally into its correct position, and the bridge had then replaced the lateral incisor.

Uneven spacing (Fig. 15.11) is also a prime indication for orthodontics. The illustrated case has

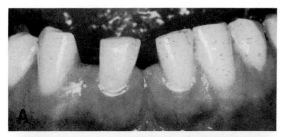

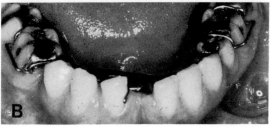

**Fig. 15.11**   Pre-bridge orthodontics. **A,** The uneven spacing caused by the loss of one central incisor would make bridgework difficult; **B,** The lateral incisor has been retracted by a simple appliance, and a three unit bridge is now straightforward.

been converted from a difficult four or five unit bridge to a simple three unit bridge.

Equilibration of precentric prematurities is desirable on those teeth which are destined for preparation. If a prematurity is removed by the preparation without knowledge of its relationship, the occlusal pattern can be changed leading to loss of occlusal clearance of the preparation (Ch. 12).

The pattern and strength of occlusal function in lateral and protrusive excursions is of great importance in anterior bridgework. For example, an upper lateral incisor can be replaced as a cantilever bridge from the canine in favourable cases. But this design should not be used if the pontic will receive lateral stresses from the lower incisors in lateral excursions. This would result in unfavourable rotational forces being applied to the canine. In these circumstances, the bridge should either have positive canine guidance, thereby discluding the lateral incisor pontic, or it should involve the central incisor as well in a fixed-fixed design (Fig. 15.12).

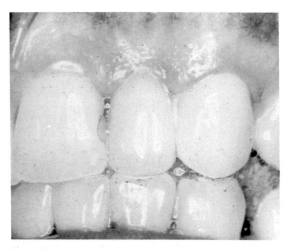

**Fig. 15.12** The |2 has been replaced as a cantilever bridge from the |3. In left lateral excursion, the pontic takes all the load and transmits this as rotational forces to the canine, which was painful. The bridge should have been made to maintain canine guidance.

### Abutment tooth assessment

The biological integrity of all the teeth must be clear from the start. Those teeth to be included in the bridge should not have pulps of dubious vitality nor have any root fillings of questionable prognosis.

Loss of periodontal support does not in itself preclude the use of particular teeth as retainers, but the disease must be controlled and stable.

These points, then, imply that a very thorough examination of the mouth aided by vitality tests and radiographs (Ch. 2) is essential prior to the prescription of bridgework.

Teeth that are provisionally designated for retainers should have any restorations of unknown origin or quality removed, and the remaining tooth examined to determine its physical and biological state. Even if the restoration's natural history is well known, it must be assessed for its possible durability under a retainer when prepared. A simple example is the replacement of a non-pinned amalgam by a pinned core because the retention of the former might well be removed during preparation (Fig. 15.13).

### Aesthetics

The provision of good aesthetics is clearly an important goal for both the patient and the continuing reputation of the clinician.

The basic design outline will detail those areas to be tooth-coloured and those to be in metal, and the patient should be aware of and approve such recommendations. Now further consideration must be given to the particular characteristics of tooth colour and position (Fig. 15.14).

The technician must be involved at this stage to give advice about any shade matching problems which might dictate a change in design or might require special techniques (Ch. 18).

If the existing tooth shape and position is satisfactory for appearance and function, then this must be copied exactly. This original blueprint may be in the form of a denture or a semi-permanent resin-retained bridge. However, if a change in aesthetics is proposed, then this needs to be clearly defined at the planning stage.

Small changes, such as the closure of a diastema, can be easily accomplished, but major changes, such as reduction of overjet, are far more complicated. This may involve elective devitalization of teeth outside the proposed arch line, together with post and cores, and, worse still, the positioning of retainers or pontics in zones where tongue activity may make these unstable.

## TREATMENT OF POTENTIAL ABUTMENT TEETH

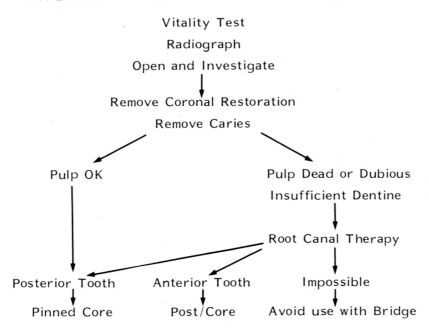

Vitality Test

Radiograph

Open and Investigate

Remove Coronal Restoration

Remove Caries

Pulp OK                                      Pulp Dead or Dubious

Insufficient Dentine

Root Canal Therapy

Posterior Tooth        Anterior Tooth        Impossible

Pinned Core            Post/Core             Avoid use with Bridge

**Fig. 15.13** The treatment of potential abutment teeth.

This type of major cosmetic change should only be attempted when the patient's objectives and motivation are clearly established, and the clinician is confident that these can be satisfied. Additional abutments will need to be included in the design to withstand the unfavourable muscle forces. In other words, it is a permanent splint that is being constructed.

The provisional restoration needs to be very accurate, and considerable time must be spent in assessing its stability. The patient must also be in absolute agreement that the new teeth are what were envisaged. Figure 15.15 shows a case where the overjet and incisor irregularity have been reduced by means of a splint. This involved devitalization of the central incisors and crown preparations on the lateral incisors and canines.

The extent of the change, particularly in overjet, was quite small and the amount of work involved was large, but the end result was patient satisfaction.

A word of warning — dentists and plastic surgeons are prone to the attention of perfection seeking individuals. If the patient appears to be

making unreasonable or strange demands, the dentist should be suspicious. In this case it is better to refuse to provide treatment, tactfully.

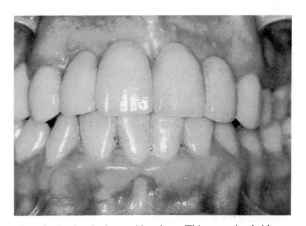

**Fig. 15.14** Aesthetic considerations. This extensive bridge replaces all the upper anterior teeth, and shows examples of characterization. Each interdental space is stained with a blue-black line, neck stains have been added to create the appearance of natural embrasures and the appearance of root dentine has been created at the necks of the central incisors.

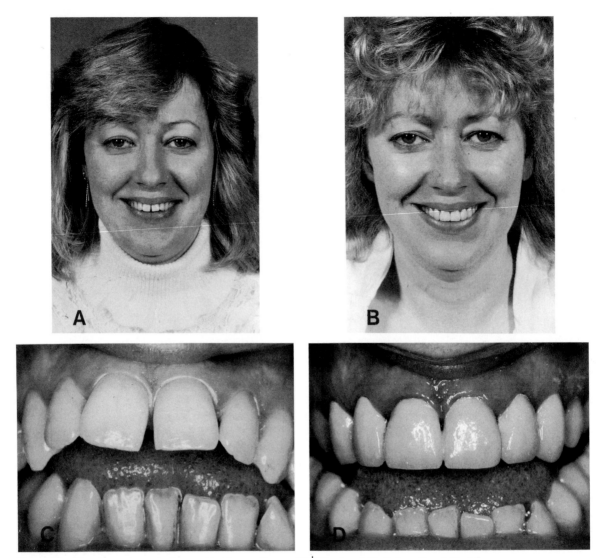

**Fig. 15.15**  The change in aesthetics provided by a splint on 321|123. **A** and **C**, Before; **B** and **D**, After.

## BASIC BRIDGE DESIGNS

Much (if not all) bridge design is empirical, based on the accumulated, acquired wisdom of clinical experience, or simple personal prejudice. Very little objective work has been carried out on the biomechanics of the subject. It is, of course, doubtful how much in the way of physical laws would be appropriate in an area which is so dependent on biological status and response. It is a truism to say that every case is different.

A few basic guidelines could be advanced, such as:

1. Keep designs as simple as possible. For example, if two upper incisors are being replaced, make two three-unit bridges, rather than one six unit;
2. Use a canine or molar wherever possible;
3. Avoid upper lateral incisors as strategic abutments.

A single upper central incisor is better replaced by a three unit cantilever from canine and lateral incisor, rather than a fixed – fixed bridge using the lateral incisor and the other central. Here, the use of the canine increases the periodontal support of the bridge and the lateral incisor is not so vulnerable.

The diagrams in Figure 15.16 show a series of

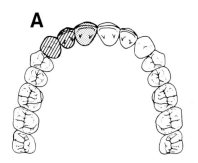

**Fig. 15.16**  Some basic bridge designs.
**A**,  Cantilever
Pontic: 1|
Retainers: 32|
Uses canine as major support.

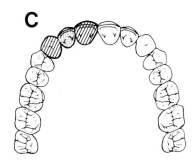

**B**,  Cantilever
Pontic: 2|
Retainer: 3|
Must be no lateral stress on pontic in excursions.

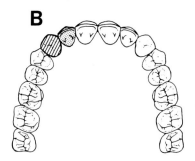

**C**,  Fixed–fixed
Pontic: 2|
Retainers: 31|
If the occlusion causes lateral stress on the pontic in B, use the central incisor as well.

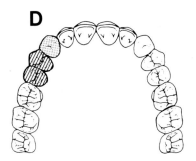

**D**,  Cantilever
Pontic: 3|
Retainers: 54|
Lateral excursion must have group function, to avoid the pontic taking lateral stress.

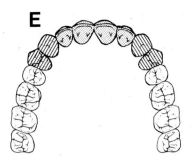

**E,**  Fixed–fixed
Pontics: 21|12
Retainers: 43|34
Root area of combined retainers provides good support.

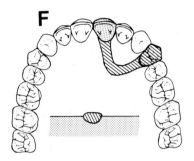

**F,**  Spring cantilever
Pontic: |1
Retainer: |4
The palate and the flexibility of the bar absorb occlusal loading on the pontic, and the premolar simply retains the bridge in place. Inset shows bar profile in the tissues.

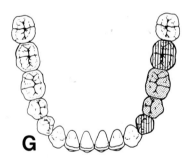

**G,**  Fixed–fixed
Pontics: ⌐56
Retainers: ⌐47
If the roots of the retainers are small, add ⌐3.

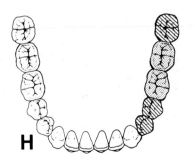

**H,**  Fixed–fixed
Pontics: ⌐67
Retainers: ⌐348
Retention of the ⌐34 preparations must be similar, otherwise uneven cement lute stresses will lead to cementation failure.

standard designs which will work in favourable cases. Unfavourable factors, such as short roots, loss of periodontal support, heavy occlusion and so on, might cause the empirical addition of a further retainer to each design. Full crowns are shown as the retainers, but partial veneer crowns could be substituted.

## PRECISION RETAINERS

Simply, these are connectors which retain dentures without the use of externally visible clasps. The denture may be a complete denture or a partial, unilateral or bilateral. The unilateral partial denture is sometimes called a removable bridge. This is considered to have an advantage over a conventional bridge in that it is partly tissue borne, and therefore larger spans can be contemplated. Again, this is an empirical decision.

Precision retainers consist of two precisely interlocking parts, a male and a female, one of which is soldered into the retaining crown and the other which is processed into the denture. The part fitting the retaining crown may be intra- or extracoronal. The intracoronal type requires a more extensive tooth preparation to accommodate it within the crown profile.

There are many designs, most named after their inventors. Some include internal springs and stress breaking devices, and others fix the denture permanently by means of minute screws. They are expensive and technically demanding to use, but do have advantages in a few particular cases. It is worth being familiar with two or three types of basic design.

The use of precision retainers in complete dentures is discussed in Chapter 19. For a unilateral space, bounded by teeth, a pair of extracoronal retainers, such as the Mini-Dalbo, can be used (Fig. 15.17).

Where there has been extensive alveolar loss, a denture base is often necessary to make up the deficiency. Where there is room in the occlusion and some splinting action is required to hold the abutment teeth, a bar type, such as the Andrews, is useful (Fig. 15.18).

Larger partial dentures may be aesthetically more pleasing in the absence of clasps, but teeth having the precision retainers on them must be splinted for support to other teeth, thus making the overall treatment plan complicated, costly and technically demanding.

## SPECIAL PROBLEMS

### Cleft palate

With modern orthodontic and plastic surgical management of the cleft palate, the cases with massive crown work to retain obturators are a thing of the past. The cases treated by modern techniques, though, may require crowning of teeth which are

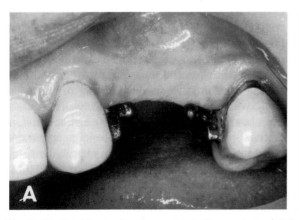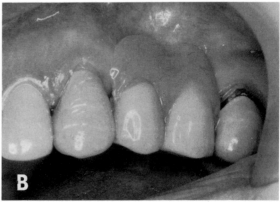

**Fig. 15.17** Precision retained removable bridge, replacing |45 from crowns on |36. **A,** Mini-Dalbo attachments on metal-ceramic crowns, in |3 and |6. **B,** The prosthesis in place.

spans of more than four units anteriorly will need a metal sub-frame and resin facings, or posteriorly will need to be all metal for durability. It may be in use for as long as six weeks and therefore needs to be constructed carefully.

Chairside construction of provisional bridges is appropriate for short spans of uncomplicated bridgework.. These may only be in place for a matter of a couple of weeks, and for this relatively short period, the inferior aesthetics and strength are not usually a problem.

### Chairside construction technique

The pre-operative model is used as a template with the shape of the pontics and retainers provided either from the diagnostic waxing or from the addition of denture teeth to the model. The areas of the buccal and palatal surfaces which are to be cut for veneers should be overcontoured by adding wax so that eventually this will be reproduced in the provisional as thicker walls. Without this, the resin overlying the veneer preparation would be too thin for adequate strength.

An impression is made of the area of the bridge in silicone putty. A sectional impression only is required, but this must extend by at least one tooth either side of the abutment teeth so that the impression, or mould as it is to become, is stabilized in the mouth. A refinement of the putty impression is to use a vacuum formed resin sheet which is moulded to the pre-operative model.

At the chairside, following the completion of the preparations, the seating of the mould is checked for accuracy, gingival retraction cord is placed to protect the gingival tissues, a smear of petroleum jelly is applied to the dentine surfaces and a selfcuring resin, preferably one designed for provisional bridges, is mixed and syringed around the necks of the prepared teeth and into the mould. The filled mould is seated onto the teeth, located correctly and left in place until the initial set of the resin has occurred. The mould is then removed together with the new bridge and its excess. The excess is trimmed carefully back to the preparation margins and the pontic gingival margins rounded. The embrasures, particularly at the cervical margins, must be cleared carefully. The bridge is replaced onto the teeth, and the marginal adaptation checked. The occlusion is then corrected using abrasive points following identification of inaccuracies with shimstock and articulating paper. Additions to the resin can be made easily as necessary (Fig. 16.1A).

### Laboratory construction technique

The *all-resin bridge* can be made by flasking the waxed trial preparations model, perhaps having incorporated denture tooth facings as appropriate, and processing in the same way as a denture. At the chairside, the fit of the bridge is likely to be inaccurate, and it will need to be relined in resin on the preparations to achieve this (Fig. 16.1B and D).

The *metal based bridge*, whether cast in silver, student's alloy or even bonding alloy, requires exactly the same technique as that required for the final restoration. It needs to be made from an impression of the finished preparations as quickly as possible, with an all-resin bridge as a very temporary intermediate restoration (Fig. 16.1C).

If the provisional bridge has been used to verify a new occlusal scheme and has been adjusted for this or for tooth shape and position, an impression of the arch including the bridge must be taken and remounted to the existing mounted opposing model. The incisal table should be re-customized.

### PREPARATIONS

Whilst each abutment will be prepared in accordance with the basic principles discussed in Chapter 13, the major consideration in the majority of bridgework is achieving a single path of insertion for the bridge.

The desired path of insertion should be decided from the diagnostic mounting using a model surveyor, and the line should be marked on the model abutments. If a non-rigid connector is to be used with different paths for each abutment, these paths can again be marked on the model.

In short span bridges, with two or three abutments, the path can usually be transferred to the mouth by eye, with extreme care being taken to keep the burs in the single path whilst cutting.

For longer spans and multiple abutments, some additional help will be necessary. Proprietary parallelometers can be bought, the simplest of which is a pair of parallel pins on an extending arm. This

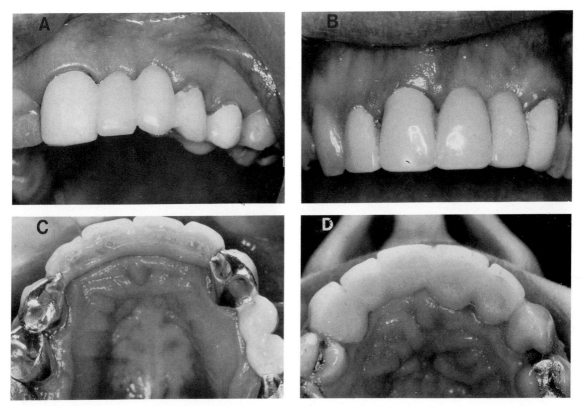

**Fig. 16.1** Provisional bridges. **A**, Cold curing resin, chairside made type. This has very bland aesthetics and has to be overcontoured for strength. It is satisfactory for short spans, or for a few days whilst a more accurate provisional is made; **B** and **D**, All resin, laboratory constructed type. The labial aspects are made from denture tooth facings and the remainder is made from a waxing and hydroflask cured acrylic. This is suitable for trying new occlusal schemes and changes in aesthetics. If it is made from trial preparations on the diagnostic mounting, the retainers will need rebasing in the mouth with the addition of cold curing resin; **C**, Cast silver/resin type. This is necessary for long spans. The incisors are denture tooth facings, retained to the metal by hydroflasked acrylic. The occlusion and aesthetics can be checked accurately on this type of provisional. This is the provisional bridge used in the case shown in Figure 15.14.

may not be sufficient for cross-arch work and some reference device can be made for the particular patient in the laboratory. A flat sheet of acrylic 2 mm thick is trimmed to fit the arch to be prepared, and modified with cold curing acrylic to locate to the occlusal surfaces accurately. It should extend beyond the buccal surfaces of the abutment teeth by about 2 mm.

The model is mounted on a surveyor whose pin is aligned with the chosen path of insertion. The acrylic sheet is placed on the model and holes are drilled by a surveyor mounted handpiece to locate pins at the side of each abutment. The pins can be screwed in, or glued by cyanoacrylate cement. This device will locate in the mouth to indicate the desired paths for each abutment.

Additional information can be provided by cutting the preparations roughly and then taking an alginate impression. This is cast in plaster mixed with hot water for a rapid set, and the resulting model checked with a surveyor for accuracy of paralleling whilst the patient remains in the chair and then has the preparations finally defined afterwards.

The presence of posts and cores in the design can be used to aid paralleling. Preparation of the posts is the first stage, and an impression is taken of the post holes. The cores can then be waxed parallel to the predicted path of insertion (Fig. 16.2), and when cemented, provide a very accurate guide for the preparation of the other abutments (Fig. 16.3).

Modification to the basic design of abutment preparations is also necessary in the connector

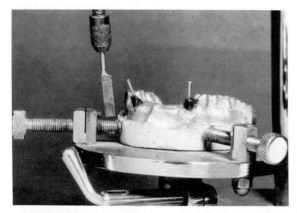

**Fig 16.2** Waxing the cores for an anterior bridge. The model has been mounted on a surveyor to align the cores precisely with the chosen path of insertion.

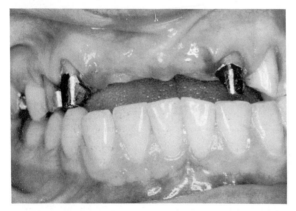

**Fig 16.3** The cores cemented. The bridge is to replace 21|1 from 43|23, and the preparations have been completed using the cores as alignment guides. Note the shape of the vital tooth preparations giving good retention and the contour allowing correct thickness of ceramic. Note also the lack of gingival trauma after preparation.

region. Tooth removal should be increased here to provide additional strength in the subsequent casting. Where precision retainers or other non-rigid connectors are to be used, box preparations will usually be necessary to accommodate them.

## IMPRESSION AND SHADE

These are dealt with in Chapters 17 and 18.

## OCCLUSAL REGISTRATION

Centric occlusion is required, with clear tooth to tooth contacts. If a position of best fit is still present,

in spite of occlusal reductions, this should be used without an inter-occlusal record; reproduction of the position from the pre-operative mounting will be possible.

If centric occlusion has been lost by the preparations, then the most accurate method of registration is by *transfer copings*. These are shells of acrylic or metal which fit the prepared teeth accurately and onto which cold curing resin is added

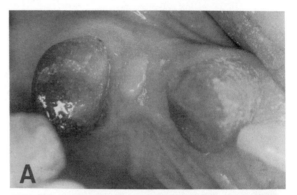

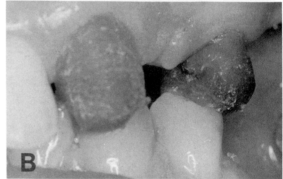

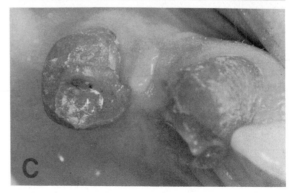

**Fig 16.4** Acrylic, laboratory made transfer copings for occlusal registration. **A**, Occlusal view; **B**, Buccal view in occlusion; **C**, Occlusal view of registration imprints. This was the registration for the bridge shown in Figure 15.9.

to register the tooth relationships (Fig. 16.4). The coping can be made on the master die and used to check that the preparation margins have been accurately reproduced. Metal, such as cast silver, is better than resin for this purpose if the margins are really questionable. Alternatively, copings can be made intra-orally on lubricated preparations by free-hand application of resin and the occlusion registered at the same time. Clearly, these cannot be used to check margins.

The master model, when completed, is mounted to the untouched opposing arch of the pre-operative mounting. A further face-bow registration is not necessary.

Articulator angles will have been determined from the diagnostic mounting, and can be set again for the master models. However, when actually constructing crowns and bridges, it is common to use condylar angles that are slightly lower than average. This has the effect of making cusp heights lower and cusp slopes shallower, and therefore the likelihood of introducing occlusal interferences unwittingly is much reduced.

Upon completion of the impression and registration, the provisional bridge should be cemented with a weak ZOE cement, or a proprietary temporary cement.

## TRY-IN

This is possibly the most critical stage, wherein the established errors are either seen and accepted, or completely missed. It depends on the level of perfection and perception of both the dentist and the technician as to what passes and what is rejected. Only the obvious needs stating, the larger the errors, the less the chances of success for the restoration.

### Metal subframe

The try-in of the metal subframe before the addition of ceramic has several advantages. The *accuracy* of the casting can be checked. If there are errors, then the time and cost of adding the ceramic to a deficient base are avoided. The *localization* between abutments can be checked and re-adjusted if necessary without jeopardizing the ceramic by resoldering. The *occlusion* can be checked and adjusted without damaging the ceramic glaze.

For short spans, where the dentist and technician are confident of the impression, then a metalwork try-in could be omitted. For longer spans there should always be one.

### Final bridge

The checklist below should be followed with teeth dried and isolated, and where possible, a pack in place to prevent loss of the bridge through the pharynx:

- Marginal adaptation of retainers
- Retention and stability
- Integrity of contact areas with adjacent uncut teeth
- Adaptation of the pontics to the soft tissues
- Occlusal relationships in centric, pre-centric and lateral excursions
- Aesthetics — colour, shape and tooth position
- Speech
- Patient approval

*Marginal adaptation*

A probe should traverse all the margins smoothly from tooth to retainer without catching. Positive edges can be trimmed back, but negatives edges are a deficiency and the retainer must be modified or remade. If the master die does not reproduce the defective margins, then a new impression of the problem abutment is needed. This can be relocated with the satisfactory dies and the new retainer soldered into the new restoration.

If the margin is reproduced on the original die, then ceramic could be added to the retainer. Soldering, though, to build out a deficient metal margin is not usually acceptable.

If the retainer is not seating onto the abutment margin, then the following should be checked:

- Fit surface of preparation — temporary cement remaining
- Fit surface of retainer — ceramic present casting excess from airblow
- Contact areas — tight, preventing seating
- Movement of abutments under provisional bridge
- Localization of retainers — one seats and the other(s) lifts off

The first four are fairly easy to overcome. Careful

inspection will reveal extraneous material and use of floss will demonstrate tight contacts.

Small tooth movements are possible whilst the provisional bridge is in place. This may be due to occlusal forces or to slight displacement by the temporary cement. Not every bridge seats home exactly at the first attempt, and small discrepancies can be overcome by 'stressing' the periodontal ligament by alternate loading and releasing.

Cotton wool rolls or a tongue spatula may be placed on the occlusal surface of the bridge, and by alternate clenching and relaxing, the patient can induce minor movements of the abutments. This only works for *small* seating problems.

Where one retainer fits and the other(s) does not seat fully, there can be a localization error. The bridge should be sectioned carefully into individual pieces with one connector being maintained to hold each pontic. Each retainer should be tried on its abutment individually (Fig. 16.5A). If each seats accurately, the new arrangement should be fixed by the addition of cold-curing acrylic in the mouth.

To stabilize the retainers for this procedure, a small amount of non-setting paste, e.g. zinc oxide in vaseline, should be applied to the retainers' fit surface (Fig. 16.5B). A non-residue, burn out acrylic is then carefully applied to the sectioned joint to stabilize it rigidly (Fig. 16.5C). The relocalized bridge is then removed, cleaned and returned to the laboratory for soldering (Ch. 18).

Failure of a sectioned retainer to seat requires a new impression after the preparation has been inspected carefully for undercuts. These may have created an impression fault not seen on the die.

### Retention and stability

The bridge should not be dependent on its cement lute for retention. Looseness may be caused by over-tapered preparations or poor adaptation of castings. If the fit of individual dies in their retainers is loose, the bridge should be remade. If the dies are tight, then an impression fault is possible; the impression should be taken again, after checking the parallelism of the preparations.

The bridge should not rock when pressure is applied to each retainer and if it does there is likely to be a casting error on an individual retainer or seating problems referred to earlier.

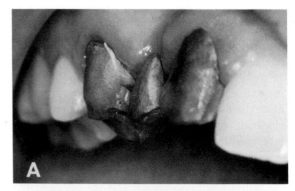

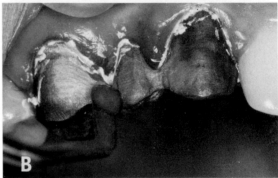

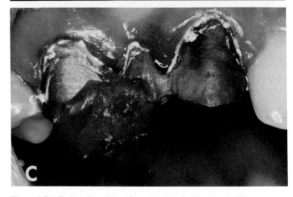

**Fig 16.5** Relocalization of a metal sub-frame. **A**, The try-in did not seat on the premolar. The bridge has been sectioned between the pontic and the premolar retainer, and now seats correctly; **B**, A zinc oxide–vaseline paste has been applied to the fitting surfaces to stabilize the bridge during application of the fluid acrylic; **C**, The acrylic must be extensive to make sure that there is no movement upon removal of the bridge and during its journey to the laboratory. This is the sub-frame for the bridge shown in Figures 12.21 and 15.10.

### Contact areas

These should be checked with floss. A correct contact allows floss to 'click' through on pressure. Slack contacts will require the addition of solder or more ceramic to correct them. Tight contacts should be eased and repolished.

### Adaptation of pontics

The soft tissue underlying a pontic should blanch slightly on insertion of the bridge. The neck of the pontic should blend smoothly with the alveolar ridge to promote natural cleaning during function (Fig. 15.14).

### Occlusal relationships

Occlusal stability should be checked by marking each new cusp/fossa relationship with articulating paper and checking that each holds shimstock on light closure. The natural cusp/fossa relationships should also be checked with shimstock to ensure that the bridge is not preventing even occlusion elsewhere.

Closure on the retruded arc of closure should be checked to ensure that the bridge is not introducing new precentric premature contacts. Cusp slopes can be adjusted but not height, as the removal of the cusp tip will also remove occlusal stability.

Lateral and protrusive excursions should be checked for freedom of movement and for the presence of non-working interferences. If the bridge is reproducing canine guidance, this must be steep enough to disclude the non-working side. If interferences are introduced, the bridge must be modified, rather than equilibrating other teeth. Similarly, incisal length should provide enough depth of incisal guidance to disclude the posterior teeth.

### Aesthetics

The patient should be the final arbiter of the appearance. Modifications to the shade are discussed in Chapter 18.

### Speech

A standard passage of prose to be read by the patient can be used, but it is better for natural speech to be the deciding factor. This means a period of trial cementation.

## TRIAL CEMENTATION

Once a bridge is cemented permanently, the modifications that can be made are very limited. Therefore, the best course is to fit the bridge with a weak temporary cement and allow the patient to try it for about four weeks for speech and function, and for the other members of the family to approve the appearance.

The patient must be warned, though, of the weakness of the cement, and to return immediately if there are any symptoms. This will usually mean cement failure in a retainer.

## PERMANENT CEMENTATION

The patient's opinion and experience of the bridge are discussed after the trial cementation, and the occlusal relationships re-checked. Modifications to tooth shape, colour and size are possible to a limited extent, and these are discussed in Chapter 18. If further modifications are made or the patient has any reservations, another period of trial cementation is indicated.

Only when all are satisfied should the bridge be cemented permanently. After the cement has set, the marginal adaptation should be checked again and excess cement cleaned from the embrasures and from under the pontics. The patient must be taught the appropriate oral hygiene procedures (Ch. 15).

## REVIEW AND RECALL

Finally, the bridge should be checked again a week or two after cementation and it should be ensured that the patient is performing the oral hygiene required and that there are no problems with this. Routine six-monthly recall should be arranged and the apical condition of all the abutments reviewed radiographically at this time. Further radiographs should be taken routinely every two years or so. Silent pulp death and apical infection are possibilities.

## ANTERIOR BRIDGEWORK

This presents the dual problems of combining aesthetics with function. It is an important part of bridgework, since the cosmetic aspect is a strong motivation factor for the patient. This, coupled with

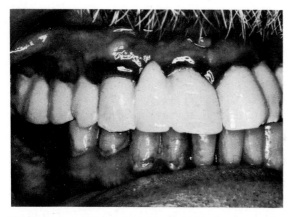

**Fig 16.6** An awful anterior bridge, which reflects no credit on the treatment planning and operative skills of the dentist or the technician. There is gross periodontal disease present, the bridge had fallen out on three occasions in its two year life, the ceramic has been poorly applied to an incorrect sub-frame design and is chipped on the incisal edges. The bridge was replaced by a partial denture.

the desire to be rid of the intrusion of a partial denture, provides a demand which can only be satisfied by the highest clinical and technical standards. The ability to make good anterior bridgework is a good practice builder; the converse is also true (Fig. 16.6).

The patient will either have a partial denture or an intermediate bridge and there are two possible lines of treatment. The existing replacement teeth may be satisfactory from the aesthetic and functional viewpoint, in which case they should be copied exactly in combination with the new retainers.

On the other hand, one or both aspects may be unsatisfactory and this will necessitate more in the way of diagnostic planning and a longer stage with the provisional bridge.

The sequence for the simple replacement of existing aesthetics and function, following stabilization is:

1. Diagnostic mounting and examination of the occlusion;
2. Customizing the incisal guidance table of the articulator;
3. Provisional bridge, preparations;
4. Provisional bridge approval;
5. Final bridge — trial cementation and permanent cementation.

Where the existing teeth and/or function are unsatisfactory, the sequence is:

1. Diagnostic mounting and examination of the occlusion;
2. Diagnostic waxing to establish new aesthetics and/or function;
3. Customize incisal guidance table to diagnostic waxing;
4. Construct provisional bridge from the above;
5. Preparations, fit provisional;
6. Check function and aesthetics of provisional, modify if necessary;
7. Approval of provisional;
8. If modifications made, impression of provisional;
9. Articulate model of approved provisional, re-customize incisal guide;
10. Mount master model, construct final bridge;
11. Trial cementation;
12. Permanent cementation.

### Case report

The principles involved in the establishment of new aesthetics and function can be illustrated by the following case. The patient requested the replacement of her existing partial denture, which had never been comfortable, by bridgework (Fig. 16.7A).

She had 32|2 missing and the decision, in principle, was to replace these teeth by two fixed–fixed bridges between 4| and 1| and |1 and |3.

The diagnostic mounting with the denture in place, showed that there were non-working interferences of the second molars on both left and right lateral excursions, leading to anterior disclusion (Fig. 16.7B & C). This was due to the denture teeth being narrow bucco-lingually and not participating in the lateral excursions; in fact, therefore, the excursions were guided by the second molar contacts, which is contrary to occlusal principles (Ch. 12).

It was decided to establish canine guidance with posterior disclusion on lateral excursions, within the framework of the existing aesthetics, which were satisfactory.

Provisional bridges were made from a diagnostic waxing which fulfilled the above objectives. These were placed in the mouth and worn for four weeks.

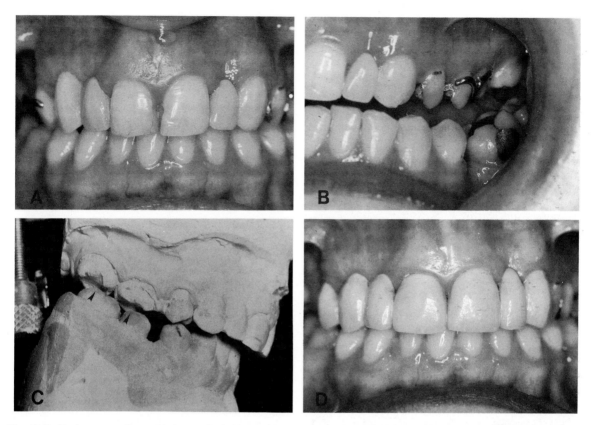

**Fig. 16.7** Replacement of a partial denture by bridgework with a change in occlusal design. **A**, 32|2 are replaced by a partial denture, which is uncomfortable; **B**, In lateral excursions, the occlusion is guided by the molars on the non-working side, leading to anterior disclusion; **C**, the diagnostic mounting shows the interferences (arrowed) on the right side; **D**, The completed bridgework — two fixed–fixed bridges, 4321| and |123, in centric occlusion.

The new occlusal scheme was comfortable and the aesthetics satisfactory. An impression of the upper arch was taken and mounted to the lower articulated cast in centric occlusion, and the incisal table customized.

To customize the incisal guide, cold-curing acrylic was placed on the incisal table, and whilst soft, the incisal pin was moved in it with the tooth to tooth contacts being maintained in protrusion and lateral excursions. When hard, the table reproduced the movement paths which were guided by the provisional bridge contours.

The master model was mounted, and the waxing of the bridge performed to reproduce the same paths. Trial cementation gave rise to no problems in four weeks and the bridges were cemented permanently (Fig. 16.7D and Fig. 16.8).

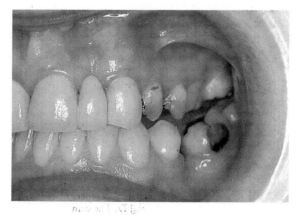

**Fig 16.8** The bridge in Figure 16.7 in left lateral excursion, showing canine guidance has been created.

## Spring cantilever bridge

In this design, the anterior pontic is retained by an abutment tooth in the posterior region and the connector is a long metal bar, which is supported by the palate (Fig. 15.16F).

The advantages of the design are that sound anterior teeth can remain uncut and that natural spacing of the anterior teeth can be reproduced. The disadvantage is the presence of the bar in the palate, which requires regular cleaning to avoid it initiating inflammation.

It is another design which has been partly superseded by resin retained bridgework, though there are still cases for which it is indicated.

The choice of abutment is important, as is the

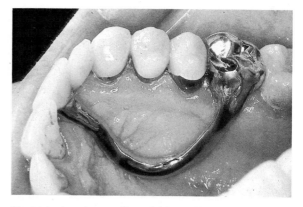

**Fig 16.9** A spring cantilever bridge retained by a molar. The premolars were not suitable because of deep caries and a questionnable prognosis.

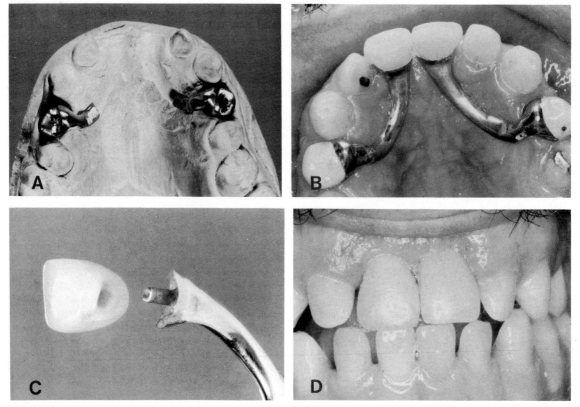

**Fig. 16.10** Two spring cantilever bridges. **A**, The working model with the metal–ceramic retainer sub-frames. The paths for the bars have been gouged from the palate at depth appropriate to the tissue compressibility. The area for the soldered joints on the retainers is some way from them, so that the ceramic will not crack when soldering takes place; **C**, Porcelain jacket crown pontic, made on an aluminous tube; **B** and **D**, The completed bridges in centric occlusion. The anterior spacing made this an ideal case for spring cantilevers.

shape of the vault of the palate. A single premolar, usually the first, is sufficient to retain the bridge, since the bar provides a tissue-borne element to the design and is also a stress breaker. A second premolar should only be incorporated if the first has a short preparation of low retention. If for any reason, the premolars are unacceptable, then the first permanent molar can be used (Fig 16.9).

The retainer can either be a partial veneer or a full crown, depending on the aesthetics, and the skill of the operator.

The palate must be shallow so that the bar is well supported. A steep vault will not support the bar and it will lie vertically, rather than horizontally, and more stress will pass to the abutment. The palate must also be 'mapped' by testing the compressibility of the tissues in the path of the bar with a ball ended instrument.

The bar should be embedded to an appropriate depth, and in the more compressible areas it should be to about 2 mm, whilst in the more fibrous areas, 0.5 mm only will be possible (Fig. 16.10A).

Figure 16.10A also shows the arrangement of two metal–ceramic crowns to link with a pair of bars. The soldered joint should be some distance from the ceramic, which will have been applied prior to soldering. Trying to solder the bar at the crown margin would almost certainly result in cracking of the ceramic.

The final bridge will require time at the fitting stage to compress the tissues under the bar before cementation. The tissue will blanch initially and tissue fluid will be displaced as the bar embeds itself. This is aided by alternate pressure and relaxation applied by the patient's masticatory muscles.

The pontic is a separate jacket crown, which can be replaced independently of the bridge if necessary in the future (Fig. 16.10C). At the fitting stage it should be left slightly long to allow for further embedding of the bar during the first week and adjusted at the review visit (Fig. 16.10D).

The patient must be shown how to clean under the bar with floss, and this procedure must be done at least once a day.

# 17. Impression techniques and materials

*G. J. Pearson*

The long chain of positive and negative dimensional pitfalls between completion of the preparation and the cementation of a cast restoration begins with the impression.

Before considering the individual groups of materials, it is important to determine the properties that are clinically desirable, both for the operator and the patient.

From the patient's viewpoint, it is desirable that the material tastes pleasant and has a short setting time. Because impression taking can be a messy procedure, the material should be easy to remove from tissues and clothes. It should not damage the oral tissues or the tooth, and very importantly, the material should not contain constituents likely to produce sensitivity reactions.

The operator's requirements are somewhat different. The material should be easy to mix with a working time that is long enough to allow it to be placed around a number of preparations before setting starts. In order to reproduce the details of the preparation, it should flow well and have a low surface tension, so that it will wet the surfaces of the preparations. The reproduction of the surface detail and the margins of the preparation is essential in order that the restoration will be a good fit and will not fail due to leakage.

Impression taking would be very easy if the materials were miscible with saliva and tissue fluid. A number of the more recently available materials do claim to be hydrophyllic, but currently the only material which does this, is the reversible hydrocolloid.

After removal from tooth undercuts, the material must have a high elastic recovery to reproduce these areas and the rate of this recovery from deformation must be rapid (Ch. 8).

The material should not be excessively rigid. If it lacks elasticity, it may well be difficult to disengage from undercuts and could traumatize the soft tissues. A stiff material will also be difficult to remove from its model and stone dies may be damaged.

Perhaps the most significant properties for clinical success are dimensional accuracy and stability. All the elastomers set by a polymerization reaction, and the crosslinking which occurs results in some shrinkage which varies with the type of material. This generally results in a contraction towards the internal surface of the impression tray, assuming the tray adhesive is strong enough to resist the forces.

With simple extra-coronal preparations this does not present major problems since the die produced from the preparation will be slightly larger than the original preparation. Therefore, the restoration will seat on that preparation, but the cement lute will be increased in width.

Greater problems exist with complex intra-coronal features, such as slots and grooves. In these cases the dimensional changes are much more complex and consequent variations result in either difficulty or failure of the restoration to seat completely.

The material should also have a high tear resistance, since once the impression has engaged in an undercut, a thin area of material may well be damaged on removal.

## IMPRESSION MATERIALS

A general classification of impression materials is given in Table 17.1. The rigid materials have fallen from grace almost completely, as have the techniques of direct wax pattern making in the mouth.

The irreversible hydrocolloids, the alginates, are excellent for preliminary impressions, but because of

**Table 17.1** Types of indirect impression materials

| Rigid | | | Elastomeric | | | |
|---|---|---|---|---|---|---|
| Composition | Hydrocolloids | | Polysulphides | Polyethers | Silicones | |
| | Irreversible | Reversible | | | Type I | Type II |
| | Alginate | Agar-agar | | | Condensation cured | Addition cured |

their dimensional instability, have no place as final impressions. The reversible hydrocolloids, e.g. agar-agar, on the other hand, are excellent for the reproduction of detail and mix well with intra-oral fluids. However, they require specialized equipment and must be cast immediately upon removal from the mouth.

The principal materials are the rubber based elastomers. Those currently available fall into three main groups, the silicones (polysiloxanes), the polysulphides and the polyethers.

The elastomers are generally available in one of four forms described as *putty*, *heavy bodied*, *regular* and *light bodied*; the basic difference between the four forms being the filler loading.

The silicone materials may be divided into two separate subgroups, *condensation curing* (Type I), and *addition curing* (Type II).

## Condensation silicones

These materials are very popular in general practice because of their clean handling and rapid set. They may come in all four consistencies, but the most popular are the putty and wash materials, the wash being light bodied. This combination is used in about 65% of all crown work in the UK. The active constituents are shown in Table 17.2.

The elastomer sets by a condensation reaction with the liberation of ethanol, which evaporates. The consequence of this is that a shrinkage of 0.5% occurs over the first 24 hours, and continues for several days. This is significant if the technical support is some distance from the practice. The greater setting contraction occurs in the light bodied materials where the elastomer is the largest component.

The light bodied material has the ability to reproduce the surface detail well, but has a relatively low tear resistance and many of the materials are difficult to handle.

The rapidity of set can lead to problems since the setting reaction is temperature dependent. There is a marked reduction in both working and setting times with a relatively small increase in ambient temperature, particularly when the humidity is high This can result in a material being placed at a time when, although it may still be manipulable, it has already commenced its setting phase. This causes the development of setting stresses in the material which will be relieved after the removal of the impression. This, in turn, will lead to a restoration which, while fitting the die, will not seat satisfactorily in the mouth. Failures with these materials are more commonly associated with complex intra-coronal preparations and bridgework.

## Addition silicones

The active constituents are shown in Table 17.2. The setting reaction here has no low molecular weight byproduct, which results in a material which shows little or no dimensional change. The shrinkage

**Table 17.2** Components of elastomeric impression materials

| Type | Base | Catalyst | Filler |
|---|---|---|---|
| Type I silicone | Dimethyl siloxane | Stannous octoate<br>Alkyl silicate | Copper carbonate or silica<br>2–8 $\mu$m |
| Type II silicone | Dimethyl siloxane | Chloroplatinic acid | Silica |
| Polyether | Polyether — ethylene imine terminated | Dichlorobenzene sulphonate | Silica |
| Polysulphide | Polysulphide (Thiokol) | Lead dioxide<br>Dibutyl phthalate | Titanium dioxide, silica, or copper carbonate |

figures quoted for these materials are in the range of 0.05–0.07% at 24 hours. However, a secondary reaction does take place if incomplete polymerization has occurred, with the liberation of hydrogen gas. A number of the materials have finely divided palladium added which is supposed to absorb the hydrogen. Because of this, impressions should not be poured immediately, otherwise the liberation of hydrogen will result in a roughened die stone surface.

The material has low tear resistance and is prone to tear if engaged in deep undercuts or if used in thin section. It is also particularly temperature sensitive.

The other main disadvantage is that the tray adhesive is not strong and is relatively unreliable. This can result in the impression material pulling away from the tray in places. This is not necessarily always visible and consequently, it is only when the restoration is tried in and does not fit that the problem becomes apparent.

The addition silicones have poor wetting characteristics and are also hydrophobic which may make model pouring troublesome.

The economics of using these materials must also be considered since they are considerably more expensive than other elastomers.

Their excellent dimensional stability often results in very accurately fitting castings which may prove difficult to seat, and the master die should be treated with the appropriate die spacer.

## Polyethers

After the condensation silicone materials, these are the most commonly used impression materials. Their components are shown in Table 17.2. They are usually purchased as a two paste system of a regular consistency.

The original materials, while apparently being very dimensionally stable, were affected by humidity and showed variable unpredictable shrinkage when a diluent paste was added. Modifications in formulation have improved this, but at the expense of the handling properties.

There have been a number of cases of allergic reactions to the material causing a burning sensation in the tissues covered by the impression and, in severe cases, marked erythema. The chemical responsible is the sulphonate ester in the catalyst, which is also used in one temporary crown and bridge material and which has also produced similar reactions in patients and staff.

The tear resistance of the material is similar to that of the silicones but its stiffness is considerably higher. This stiffness can result in problems in the laboratory, since it is relatively easy to damage the dies on removal of the impression, particularly if they are narrow. Lower incisor crown preparations can be a particular problem. For the same reason it is advisable to have a double spaced special tray so that there is more material to 'give' to facilitate the removal of the impression.

The material is quite temperature sensitive and may set rapidly on a hot day. This may be critical since the working and setting times of these materials are the fastest of all the elastomers.

## Polysulphides

These are the oldest of the elastomers and because of their reliability and strength, and in spite of their smell and dirty handling, are still used extensively.

The material is usually used as a combination of heavy and light consistencies, with the heavy bodied version particularly difficult to mix. There is also a regular consistency material. The components are shown in Table 17.2. It is the lead dioxide which makes the material unpleasant to use.

On the plus side, the material has a much higher tear resistance than the other three elastomers, but it does not show such good recovery from deformation. There is a small setting contraction of between 0.13–0.25% at 24 hours, with little further shrinkage after this. The working and setting times are the longest of all the elastomers and it appears to be the least sensitive to temperature changes.

It is fair to say that there is no ideal impression material. Each elastomer requires a slightly different technique which, once mastered, provides reliable results.

## IMPRESSION TECHNIQUES

### Management of the gingival tissues

This, and excellent control of saliva, is the key to successful impression taking.

The first requirement is that the tissues should be in good health and undamaged. Careless preparation, with abraded gingivae, will repay the operator with a poor impression. Poorly fitting provisional restorations will accumulate plaque and cause gingival enlargement and bleeding.

If there are problems, then the impression should be abandoned, accurately fitting provisionals placed, perhaps cemented with a periodontal· dressing material, and the impression taken on a subsequent visit.

## Gingival retraction

To provide clear definition of the finishing line, the gingival tissues must displaced from the preparation and any exudate from the crevice controlled. There are several types of material which may be used for this.

Mechanical displacement using a variety of cord is probably the most popular. It comes in two forms, braided and twisted (Fig. 17.1). The braided form is easier to place but is usually quite thick since it is made up of three or four strands. The twisted type is finer but has a tendency to become untwisted during placement.

There are also a number of elasticated rings which may be pushed over the preparation and into the crevice.

All the proprietary brands may be impregnated with agents to control oozing from the crevice; these may be *vasoconstrictors* or *styptics*. Epinephrine (adrenaline) hydrochloride is the most common of the first group, but must be avoided in certain patients who have either cardiovascular problems or are

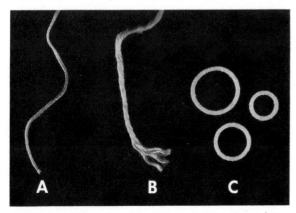

**Fig. 17.1** Gingival retraction cords. **A**, braided; **B**, twisted; **C**, elasticated rings.

sensitive to it. Aluminium trichloride, alum, is a common styptic. As well as being impregnated in the cord, both may be purchased as liquid solutions. Care must be exercised in their use, since excess application can cause irreversible damage to the tissues.

***Cord placement.*** Care must be taken in placement of the cord otherwise damage will occur to the epithelial attachment. The cord is laid around the tooth which must be isolated by cotton wool rolls and a saliva ejector. The width of the cord should match the depth of the crevice, and if necessary, a multi-stranded cord can be split into several thin strands. It is better, though, to have cords of different diameters available.

The cord is pressed gently into the gingival crevice using a small flat plastic instrument, keeping the cord between the blade and the tissue. A local analgesic is often advisable as the procedure can be uncomfortable.

The cord should not be left in situ too long since permanent recession may be caused. About five minutes is necessary to provide optimum retraction, maintaining saliva control all the time.

If the cord does not obstruct the margins of the preparation, it can be left in place whilst the impression is taken. If this technique is used, it is most important to remember to remove the cord before the patient leaves the surgery. To remove the cord, it should be first moistened with water or the friable gingival tissue may be damaged. It is more common, though, to remove the cord when the impression material is ready to syringe around the preparation. The cord must be removed very gently to prevent the initiation of bleeding or oozing.

It is sometimes possible to dispense with retraction and blow the light bodied material into the gingival crevice with compressed air. This is quite effective, but may result in a very thin section of rubber because of the lack of retraction, and this is liable to distort or tear.

## Electrosurgery

This technique involves the use of a high frequency electric current which may be used to either *coagulate* bleeding tissues or *fulgurate* (spark drying by ionization). When used carefully, it can produce a very clearly defined margin.

There is a risk, however, that the misuse of this technique will result in serious gingival tissue damage, particularly if the tissues are inflamed and oedematous at the time of surgery. Its main advantage is the haemostasis obtained.

### Special trays

The main advantage of a correctly made special tray is that it ensures that the thickness of the impression material is uniform, thereby reducing risk of uneven distortion. The tray will also confine the material, assist in its adaptation to the teeth and prevent it escaping into the rest of the mouth.

Adequate spacing should be provided between the tray and the teeth to accommodate a reasonable volume of impression material and stops should be placed around the arch to ensure that the tray locates accurately onto the teeth. It should be extended to about 2 mm below the gingival margin of all teeth and should wrap around the end of the alveolar ridge to confine the material to the tray. It must be made of a rigid material which will not flex or distort (Fig. 17.2).

The weak link may be the tray adhesive. Those used for the polysulphides are very good, but those provided for the addition silicones are poor and perforations should be incorporated in the tray to assist retention.

Whichever type is used, it must be given adequate time to dry before the material is mixed; this may be as much as 15 minutes.

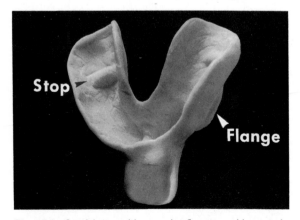

**Fig. 17.2** Special tray with posterior flanges to aid removal and occlusal stops to locate it on the teeth.

Full arch, rather than sectional, impressions are desirable for accuracy of occlusal contacts.

### Handling the materials

There are three main ways in which impression materials may be used:

- Putty and wash
- Regular/universal single mix
- Light and heavy bodied double mix

### Putty and wash technique

This technique uses a very high consistency putty within a stock tray instead of a special tray, together with a fluid, light bodied corrective or perfecting wash.

Condensation and addition silicones are the only successful materials that have been produced for this technique. There have been a number of poly-sulphide putty materials, but they have proved unacceptable.

The technique has the possible advantage that no special tray is required, but there are dangers of uneven shrinkage setting up stresses within the material. The later release of the stresses leads to dimensional inaccuracies.

Putty and wash materials may be used in one stage or two stage techniques.

**One stage.** Here, both the putty and wash materials are fluid at the same time. Following mixing, the perfecting paste is syringed around the preparation, ensuring that the nozzle of the syringe remains within the exuding material to reduce the risk of air blows, beginning at the distal margin of the preparation and working forward (Fig. 17.3). It is necessary to cover the preparation and the occlusal surfaces of the adjacent teeth with a thin film to avoid distortions.

The putty is loaded into a rigid stock tray as soon as the syringe has been filled, and is inserted into the mouth immediately the wash is in place. All these materials are very rapid setting and working time is exceptionally short.

Considerable pressure will be required to seat the tray because of the stiffness of the putty. The tray and impression material must be supported under moderate pressure until the materials have set.

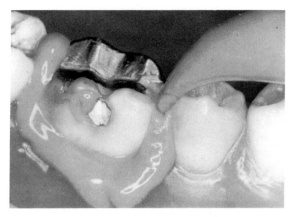

**Fig. 17.3** Syringing the light bodied material around the gingival margin. Care must be taken to apply the material to the tooth surface so that air does not become trapped.

Disturbances at this stage may well result in the impression dragging and distorting.

It is essential that the tray is rigid, otherwise it will flex under the pressure required for seating. On removal it will return to its unflexed state and this in turn will result in a distorted impression. The other problem which can occur with this technique is that the excessive pressure may result in displacement of the perfecting material away from the preparation. This results in a lack of detail where it is most needed.

**Two stage.** Here the putty 'tray' is prepared before the wash is mixed. The stock tray is first filled with the putty and seated home. A polyester sheet may be placed as a spacer on the surface of the putty before insertion, or, alternatively, the tray may be rocked to provide the space necessary for the wash.

Once the putty has set it is removed, washed and sluice ways cut in the buccal and lingual aspects in the areas adjacent to the preparation. Any material remaining approximally is also removed. The putty must be clean and dry.

The perfecting wash is syringed around the preparation and all occlusal fissures to form a thin film over the area where fine detail is required. The putty 'tray' is then reseated and the wash and putty will unite chemically as the wash sets.

The results using this technique can be good but a number of problems may arise:

- Saliva interposed between the putty and wash
- Build up of perfecting material in certain parts of the occlusal section of the impression which results in an incorrect occlusal relationship. This usually follows inadequate sluice way preparation in the primary putty impression
- Displacement and distortion of the tray during its second seating. This can result in uneven distribution of the wash and, worse, distortion of the tray itself

*Special tray technique*

The putty/wash techniques involve the production of a close fitting 'tray' in putty, but this is bulky and can introduce errors with incorrect seating. A special tray saves impression material and is easier to handle.

**Two mix technique.** The materials used are light and heavy bodied with the the heavy bodied material acting as a support for the fine detail reproducing light bodied material. The light bodied material is syringed around the preparation and onto the occlusal surfaces of the other teeth, and the heavy bodied material is loaded into the special tray which is seated with a puddling movement. The puddling reduces the risk of air incorporation within the material mass.

In the upper arch, the tray should be seated distally first and then rotated to bring the anterior portion into place. This prevents the material tracking down the pharynx.

The tray must be located accurately and held immobile until the material has set.

If the tray is not placed as soon as the light bodied material has been syringed, there is a risk of saliva contamination between the materials and impression failure. Impressions of the lower molars are the most vulnerable, with the tongue often interposing at the crucial stage.

This problem may be reduced by not introducing the light bodied material until the heavy bodied material is almost mixed. However, too much delay may mean handling the material beyond the point when it has commenced its setting phase.

Quite heavy pressure should be applied for about the first 15 seconds after insertion to ensure that the material flows, and, at the same time, it is important to ensure that the stops on the fit surface of the special tray locate accurately on the surfaces of the teeth. Without the stops, the tray will come into contact with tooth surface over a large area, and even in the area of the preparation, with a consequent failure of the impression.

*Single mix technique.* The special tray technique may be used with materials of a single, regular, or medium bodied consistency using the same mix in both the tray and the syringe. Whilst this can be successful, it is sometimes difficult to syringe the material because it is stiffer than the light bodied type, and the tray portion can flow rather freely because it is more fluid than the heavy bodied type.

### Removal of the impression

It is always tempting to remove the impression as soon as the outer aspect of the material has set. This may have disastrous consequences, as the light bodied materials set at a slower rate than the heavy bodied materials.

Early disturbance of the materials will result in the distortion of the impression and dragging of the material at the margins of the preparation.

The best indication that the material has set in the mouth is when the material has set on the mixing pad, and a timer may give some guidance. Ambient temperature and humidity cause large deviations from manufacturer predicted behaviour, and it is better to leave the material in place for as long as possible.

The impression should be removed with the minimum of rocking or shaking. One sharp pull in the line of insertion of the preparations is the ideal. This is assisted by having flanges at the side of the special tray, rather than using the handle.

### Assessment of impressions

After removal, the impression should be thoroughly washed to remove all contaminants and then dried. Careful examination should made in good light, using a hand lens if necessary. The operating light or fibre optic illumination is usually suitable.

A clear outline of the finishing margin all round the preparation should be visible with a small extent of impression material beyond it (Fig. 17.4).

There should be no air blows on the the margin but sometimes *small* air blows on the fit surface may be accepted (Fig. 17.5). Subsurface air voids may not be seen and a special check is necessary (Fig. 17.6). This may be done by gently pushing the surface of the

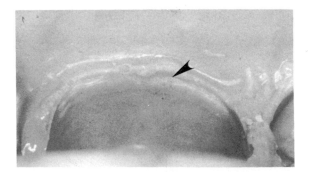

**Fig. 17.4** An impression of a chamfer finishing line (arrowed). Clarity is essential here for the technician to be able to see where to finish the waxing. There should be registration of uncut tooth beyond the finishing line.

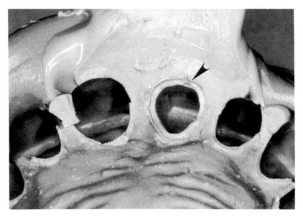

**Fig. 17.5** An impression of a shoulder. The air-blow (arrowed) does not obstruct the edge of the finishing line, and therefore the impression can be used. The technician will have to trim the defect away on the die.

material with a round ended instrument. Any areas where the surface indents indicate that there are large air voids beneath which would only become apparent on pouring the model (Fig. 17.7).

Care should be taken to ensure that the impression has not been contaminated by saliva. This is usually apparent as glazed surface with a loss of definition on the preparation. Blood entrapment is indicated by a bubbling of the surface in the area of the contamination.

Finally it is important to ensure that the material has not pulled away from the tray. This should be apparent at the periphery of the impression where it is easy to see.

If there is any doubt about the accuracy of the

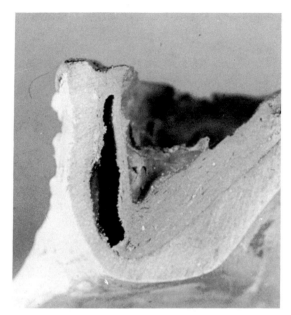

**Fig. 17.6** Large sub-surface air void under the impression of the preparation. On casting, the die stone displaced the thin layer, and the die had a surface bulge on it. The fault arose due to poor loading of the tray.

impression, it may be possible to pour it immediately and examine the preparations.

This may save time and money, but should be done in liaison with the technician, to ensure that the appropriate casting technique is used.

## SUMMARY

In order to achieve an adequate impression the following check list should be considered:

1. Special tray;
2. Choose appropriate materials;
3. Gingival tissues — healthy, no excessive bulk;

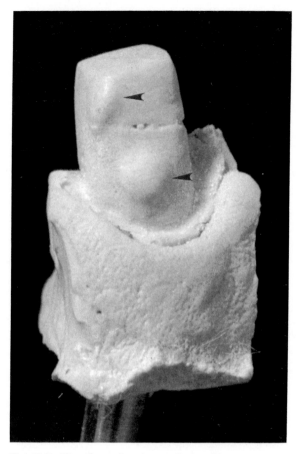

**Fig. 17.7** Two die artefacts (arrowed) caused by stone displacing light bodied material into sub-surface voids.

4. Margins of preparation clearly defined;
5. Isolate — must be clean and dry;
6. Gingival retraction — just subgingival;
7. Handle materials correctly;
8. Impression free from contamination, airblows etc.

# 18. Laboratory procedures

*R. J. Garn   R. Huggett*

Over the past decade, dental technicians have faced an increasing demand from clinicians for a service that offers the latest in materials and technological development. This requires not only mechanical skills and artistic ability, but also an understanding of oral anatomy, aesthetics, chemical and physical properties of the materials and design features.

Collaboration between the clinician and the technician, which includes clear and precise communication and respect for the role that each plays, leads to greater efficiency and is vital to the success of any laboratory constructed restoration.

## DIAGNOSTIC AND TREATMENT PLANNING PROCEDURES

The diagnostic mounting (Ch. 12) is invaluable for the discussion of a treatment plan with the laboratory. Design, aesthetics, types of materials to use and an indication of final cost can all be considered. Angulation of abutment teeth will affect the path of insertion of a bridge and it should be assessed with a parallelometer or surveyor in the laboratory. Telescopic crowns or movable joints may be necessary to overcome difficulties of alignment.

Diagnostic waxing can be used to demonstrate the repair of chipped teeth and diastema closure, illustrate contour, restored outline form and, of course, a complete redesign of the occlusion. The clinician and the patient are thereby given the opportunity to consider the proposed plan so that the objectives are clearly defined for all parties.

### Choice of materials

This will be governed by a number of factors including the size of the restoration, the availability of space and an estimate of the forces likely to be applied in function.

Single casting of multiple units has been made possible by advances in materials, and this avoids the need for several soldered joints which were previously necessary. Modern semi-precious and non-precious alloys are ideal for single units and long span bridges alike.

Ceramic is the major aesthetic facing material, but where flexure of a bridge is predicted, it may be better to use a lower modulus polymeric material to avoid cracking. Developments in composite resins, involving light curing, plus heat and/or pressure, have resulted in higher strength materials which may be used for veneering a metal sub-frame. The initial aesthetics of these are excellent, but they are not proven in the long term, and are not suitable for cusp replacement.

*Ceramic bonding alloys*

These alloys should have:

- A sufficiently high melting point so that they do not deform during firing of the ceramic
- A thermal coefficient compatible with ceramic to avoid fracture on cooling after firing
- Capacity to bond chemically with the ceramic veneer

There are three main categories of alloy:

- Precious
- Semi-precious
- Non-precious

Precious metal alloys contain a large amount of gold and platinum and exhibit good bonding characteristics, are relatively easy to cast, and finish to a high lustre. Their disadvantages are high cost and their tendency to sag during firing of the ceramic, particularly when long span bridges are involved.

The semi-precious alloys have better sag resistance and consist principally of silver and palladium, with a variable amount of gold. The silver sometimes leads to 'greening' of the ceramic if the alloy has been overheated during casting and is visible at the metal–ceramic junction.

Both precious and semi-precious alloys have small traces of base metals, (iron, indium, tin or zinc), which oxidize on firing to form a film which bonds chemically with the ceramic.

Non-precious, or base metal, bonding alloys are either nickel–chromium or cobalt–chromium. They are cheap, but more difficult to cast, and harder to finish. Their high modulus of elasticity gives them the highest sag resistance of all the bonding alloys. The nickel and the chromium oxidize on firing to form the oxide layer for bonding. However, this can be uncontrolled, and was one of the major limitations of the early alloys.

Small amounts of beryllium are present in some alloys and this is poisonous. The technician must take care not to inhale the dust whilst grinding the casting. In addition, there are some reservations about the inclusion of nickel, which may induce a sensitivity reaction in patients.

**Bonding mechanism.** This depends on three factors:

- Chemical — during firing an oxide film is formed on the metal which bonds with the ceramic
- Mechanical — surface irregularities on the casting provide a key for interlocking with the ceramic
- Compressive — there is a slight mismatch between the thermal coefficients of expansion of the ceramic and the alloy. That of the ceramic is higher so that on cooling the ceramic shrinks very slightly more and grips the metal. A curved surface is necessary for this to happen

The integrity of the final restoration is dependent upon good preparation design and attention to detail during construction.

**Planning the laboratory stages**

The discussion of the diagnostic models will have led to an agreed design for the crowns, bridges or dentures. The provision of metal or ceramic occlusal surfaces will have been decided, and the clinician must make sure that the preparations conform to this. Factors that may have to be considered include the provision of rest seats, the making of space to accommodate precision retainers and the path of insertion of a bridge.

Detailed planning must also occur on the sequence of appointments, the requirements at each, and the time the laboratory will need to construct each stage. Will there be a metal-work try-in, a try-in of the unglazed ceramic or a session devoted to staining and characterization? How will the occlusion be registered?

All this is essential for a smooth progression of the case. A rough outline of the general stages involved in a typical case is given below:

**Clinic:** Clinical examination and radiographs; diagnostic impressions, facebow and occlusal records; record shade;
**Laboratory:** Cast diagnostic models and duplicate; articulate and survey. Discuss case with clinician and agree design and stages; prepare provisional crowns/bridges as necessary; construct special trays;
**Clinic:** Discuss design with patient; confirm articulation; tooth preparations and impressions; occlusal record; fit provisionals;
**Laboratory:** Cast and articulate working models; wax, invest and cast metalwork; assemble for soldering;
**Clinic:** Metalwork try-in — check occlusion, contacts and margins;
**Laboratory:** Add ceramic, characterize;
**Clinic:** Fit restorations — check occlusion, contacts and margins; check shade;
**Laboratory:** Adjust shade, reglaze and repolish:
**Clinic:** Cementation.

## PREPARATIONS

### Veneer crowns

The chamfer finishing line provides a definite margin for finishing purposes and is conservative of tooth tissue. A clearance of at least 1 mm occlusally in centric and all excursions is essential. The shape of the reduction should conform to the original occlusal form to aid the technician in the placement of cusps.

The buccal reduction should also follow the original tooth contour so that an even thickness of restoration is provided without either over-contouring, or thinning the casting to keep proper anatomy.

### Porcelain jacket crown

Because of the brittleness of porcelain, a full shoulder 1 mm wide is essential to allow the laboratory to make a crown of consistent strength. A long preparation will support the porcelain throughout its profile, but a short one can initiate an area of stress in the palato-gingival area leading to the classic semi-lunar fracture.

All line and point angles should be gently rounded because sharp angles make the adaptation of platinum foil difficult and also lead to stress concentrations in the porcelain.

### Metal–ceramic crowns

The majority of technical problems arise because of insufficient clearance of either the buccal face or, where ceramic has been prescribed for the occlusal surface, inadequate clearance there.

In order to accommodate ceramic and metal cervically, a 1.5 mm shoulder is required. This permits 1 mm of ceramic and 0.5 mm of metal sub-frame. Ideally, 2 mm is necessary to accommodate ceramic on the occlusal surface, to provide strength to resist occlusal loads. However, the occlusal surface is easier to make in metal for accurate occlusal stops, and this should be discussed at the planning stage. Figures 18.1 and 18.2 show the various designs of sub-frame that may be used.

The ceramic must be supported by metal throughout, and be of an even thickness for colour consistency. An inadequate reduction will result in an overcontoured crown with good colour but poor gingival condition (Fig. 18.3).

When waxing the sub-frame for a metal–ceramic bridge, the technician will be concerned with achieving the maximum light transmission consistent with the support for the ceramic. The palatal collar has the dual purpose of supporting ceramic and resisting distortion as it extends into the connector region (Fig. 18.4). It must be free of the gingivae approximately to allow good cleaning and gingival health (Fig. 18.5).

The sub-frame should allow an even 1 mm of ceramic throughout for shade control and strength. The metal–ceramic interface must be smooth and gently rounded to prevent stress concentrations. Lateral excursions should be checked to ensure that

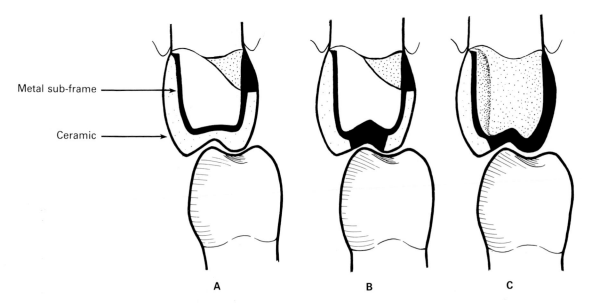

Metal sub-frame

Ceramic

A                    B                    C

Fig. 18.1   Variations in the metal sub-frame design for metal ceramic crowns on posterior teeth. **A**, Occlusal surface in ceramic; **B**, 'Island' metal centric stop; **C**, Occlusal surface and palatal cusp in metal — *preferred design*.

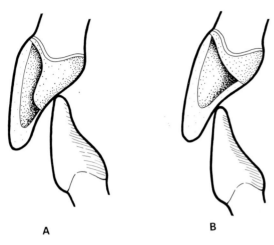

**A**                    **B**

**Fig. 18.2** Variations in metal sub-frame design for metal–ceramic crowns on anterior teeth. **A**, Centric stop and some anterior guidance in metal–*preferred design*; **B**, Most of palatal surface in ceramic.

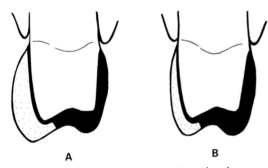

**A**                    **B**

**Fig. 18.3** The consequences of an under-reduced preparation for a metal-ceramic crown. **A**, The crown is made bulbous to reproduce the correct shade; **B**, The correct contour is reproduced, but this means that the ceramic is too thin and a poor shade is the result.

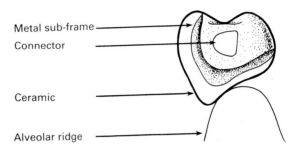

Metal sub-frame
Connector
Ceramic
Alveolar ridge

**Fig. 18.4** Bucco-lingual section through a lower premolar pontic. The metal extends from the cusp into the connector region and has a broad area of attachment, with most of the embrasure being metal also. Ceramic occupies the gingival surface and just touches the ridge buccally. The occlusal width is the same as that of the tooth it replaces.

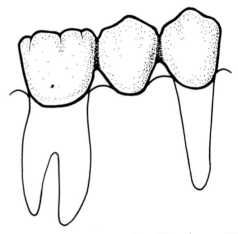

**Fig. 18.5** The premolar pontic has wide embrasure spaces on the gingival aspect to allow cleaning.

the interface on the occlusal surface does not receive occlusal loads. If a premolar, for example, is involved in group function, then the metal should be extended to receive the whole functional path.

In bridgework, fatigue of the connectors can be avoided by increasing the clearance of the preparations in the pontic areas.

**Common errors**

From the laboratory viewpoint, the following are common sources of restoration failure:

- Non-correction of occlusal problems
- Poorly shaped preparation — no retention; no ceramic support; insufficient shoulder
- Undercut preparation leading to stress
- Incorrect choice of material

## IMPRESSIONS AND MODELS

These have been discussed from the clinical viewpoint in Chapter 17. The laboratory should always be informed of the type of impression material used so that the production of the working die is done correctly. For example, addition cured silicones may release hydrogen if cast too soon, and this will affect the model surface. If metal plated models are required, the process will be affected by the impression type.

# 19. Tooth surface loss

*P. H. Jacobsen*

Tooth surface loss refers to the results of the interrelated effects of attrition, abrasion and erosion. *Attrition* is the loss of enamel and dentine that results from tooth to tooth contact; *abrasion* implies the introduction of a third body — an abrasive agent — between or against the tooth surface, and *erosion* implies a chemical aetiological agent. The effects of these factors may be accelerated by several other aspects, which include:

- Developmental anomalies of the enamel and dentine, e.g. amelogenesis imperfecta
- Posterior tooth loss, resulting in chewing being moved anteriorly
- Parafunctions and habits
- Misapplication of restorative materials
- Dietary imbalance
- Systemic disease

As teeth are retained into old age, so the natural occurrence of surface loss has become more common.

## AETIOLOGY AND CLINICAL FEATURES

### Developmental anomalies

Localized enamel *hypoplasia* is never a serious problem since isolated zones of surface loss will not usually disturb occlusal stability.

However, the more difficult conditions are those of *amelogenesis imperfecta* and *dentinogenesis imperfecta*. These are part of a range of pathology, including osteogenesis imperfecta, which are manifestations of disturbances in the formation of calcified tissues. These disturbances are genetic in origin and are often seen as familial traits.

In amelogenesis imperfecta, the enamel matrix formation is disturbed, with normal calcification of what does form. The extent of the disorder varies from localized ares of pitting, to a very thin shell of enamel. The enamel is hard but may be deposited in fine lamellations as well as in normal prismatic structure in other areas. The teeth are poor aesthetically and vulnerable to caries and attrition in affected areas.

Dentinogenesis imperfecta is uncommon and is due to defective odontoblastic activity. The dentine is soft with the deeper layer having few tubules and incomplete calcification. Also, the pulp chamber becomes obliterated. Clinically, the weak bond of the enamel to the dentine results in enamel loss, even though the enamel itself is usually normal. The colour of the teeth is abnormal, being brownish and the roots may be stunted. Apical infection may occur because of the obliteration of the root canals.

### Posterior tooth loss

If several posterior teeth are lost, mastication is likely to be affected on the remaining anterior teeth. These teeth are not well suited to grinding movements and rapid surface loss can result. This type of problem is more common in geographic areas where the level of dental care and awareness has been inadequate, and is usually coupled with non-provision of, or refusal to wear, dentures.

Even with partial dentures present, there is a great tendency to use the natural teeth, and part of the education of the patient at the fitting stage of the dentures should be to stress the need to use them effectively.

Cases exhibit progressive loss of incisor and canine crown length, coupled with saucerization of the exposed dentine. The unsupported enamel around the 'saucer' eventually breaks off and the patient is prompted to seek treatment (Fig. 19.1).

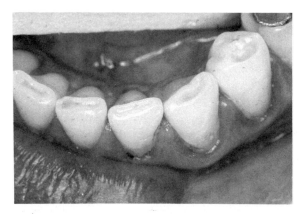

**Fig. 19.1**    Saucerized lower anterior teeth. Loss of the incisal edge enamel has led to more rapid dentine loss, and hollows in the incisal edges.

## Parafunctions and habits

*Bruxism* (Ch. 20) is the most dangerous parafunction, with enamel and dentine loss. Again, the incisor length loss is what prompts the request for treatment, but prevention, in the form of an occlusal splint, should be applied as soon as the surface loss is noted.

The exposed dentine may be sensitive, but since the attrition is usually coupled with secondary dentine formation and the retreat of the pulp, it is more often symptomless. The obliteration of the root canals by secondary dentine can lead to apical infection and the routine use of apical radiographs in the diagnostic phase is important. Root canal therapy would be indicated *before* the canals become obstructed.

Habits, such as nail biting, pipe smoking, hair grip opening and so on, can cause abnormal wear patterns, particularly of an isolated nature.

## Misapplication of restorative materials

Conventional composites and unglazed dental ceramics can remove enamel quite successfully during normal function, with their effect greatly accelerated by parafunction. Again, correct treatment planning, or early intervention, is the best course.

Coarse-particled composites should be avoided for large restorations. If a porcelain occlusal surface has been prescribed (in spite of the advice given in Chapter 12) this should be reglazed following adjustments, rather than 'polished'.

The creep of dental amalgam (Ch. 8) represents a loss of occlusal stability due to surface deformation and the upshot of this may be to put an extensively restored case into the same treatment planning group as surface loss cases.

## Dietary imbalance

High consumption of acidic food and drinks such as citrus fruits, cola and other fizzy drinks removes surface enamel. The labial aspects are usually affected, unless drinking is via a straw, in which case the palatal aspects of the upper incisors may dissolve. The worst cases are 'diet freaks' who eat large amounts of citrus fruit and brush their teeth immediately afterwards. The acid removes the mineral and the brushing removes whatever matrix is left — thus accelerating the process.

Prevention via dietary advice is the best approach, and patients could be advised to rinse with fresh water after eating fruit, rather than brushing. A reduction in intake of fruit and acidic drinks should also be advised.

The surface enamel looses its lamellated appearance and will have a high amorphous gloss. Eventually, dentine will be exposed in the eroded areas, particularly bucco-cervically and occlusally. Because the erosion causes a more rapid enamel loss than that caused by attrition alone, secondary dentine does not form quickly enough to prevent sensitivity (Fig. 19.2).

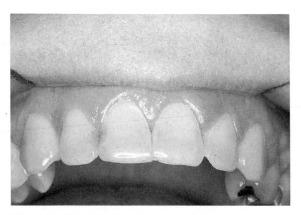

**Fig. 19.2**    Labial erosion of the upper incisors and canines. The patient was obsessed with a fresh fruit diet and tooth brushing. There is loss of much enamel with absence of lamellae, with the dentine showing through and consequent sensitivity.

## Systemic disease

Childhood diseases may interfere with the enamel mineralization of developing teeth and these may erupt with bands or localized zones of hypomineralization. These areas will be weak and, if in functional relationship with opposing teeth, will be lost fairly rapidly. The zones or bands will be chalky white and rough; they will be more prone to staining than the adjacent enamel.

In the adult, the most common systemic problem affecting the tooth surface is *gastric reflux*. Due to cardiac sphincter problems, gastric secretions are forced up the oesophagus and into the mouth. These secretions are highly demineralizing and the areas most commonly affected will be the palatal surfaces of the upper teeth. Occlusal surface loss also occurs leading to existing restorations being left above the level of the surrounding tooth. This is a classic feature of erosion in the absence of occlusal forces, where the affected tooth surface has no occlusal contact. Prolonged vomiting may also create the same picture, and is one hazard of pregnancy.

## INDICATIONS FOR TREATMENT

Cases with tooth surface loss will require restorative treatment if there is:

- Associated pathology, e.g. caries, apical infection
- Sensitivity
- Loss of occlusal stability and function
- Aesthetic problems

## PRINCIPLES OF TREATMENT

Where there is a clear external aetiological agent, this should be eliminated prior to restorative work. Correction of bad habits, dietary advice for citric acid erosion, medical referral for gastric reflux and occlusal splints for bruxism fall under this heading.

Provision of partial dentures to provide posterior support prior to the consideration of advanced restorations for worn anterior teeth is essential. A complicated treatment plan will fail if the patient will not wear the dentures.

Patients with progressing anterior surface loss, particularly males, may only be concerned that the condition does not worsen. Timely provision of partial dentures coupled with glass ionomer cement restoration of incisal edge 'saucers' may well be sufficient in many cases.

Application of desensitizing agents for patients with dentine sensitivity of occlusal surfaces may not be successful. There seems to be a difference between the response of a relatively localized zone of cervical dentine and the larger area of occlusal exposed dentine. This is particularly true of acid erosion cases where the dentinal tubules will be opened by demineralization.

Localized hypomineralized areas of enamel can be successfully restored with acid etch retained composite. Larger areas with aesthetic problems will require veneers or crowns, and those with occlusal functional problems will require onlays or crowns.

In treatment planning the more extensive case, the decisions are influenced by the age of the patient and the number of missing teeth. In the younger adult patient with an intact dentition, the indications are likely to lead to multiple crowns and ultimately to a full mouth rehabilitation (Fig. 19.3).

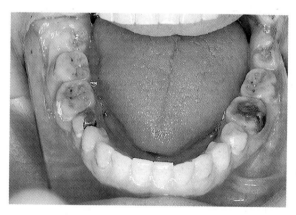

**Fig. 19.3** Posterior surface loss in a young adult. The lower incisors were the only teeth relatively unaffected.

In the older patient with many missing teeth, a transition from partial dentures to over-dentures is the better course of action.

The grey area between the two extremes of decision making depends on economic factors and the skill of the dentist. Complex treatment involving partial dentures, root canal therapy and crowns is quite possible, but patient assessment must be thorough.

## MULTIPLE CROWNS AND FULL MOUTH REHABILITATION

This very expensive and technically demanding line of treatment should not be embarked upon without first discussing the procedures and their implications with the patient, and unless the dentist has the necessary clinical training and skills to provide work of a high standard.

The sequence of treatment is as follows:

1. Stabilize active disease and eliminate surface loss aetiological agent.
   Establish excellent plaque control.
   Provide intermediate (pre-crown) restorations including dentures if necessary;
2. Advanced pre-operative phase;
3. Patient discussion, education and agreement;
4. Diagnostic splint;
5. Determine anterior guidance;
6. Restore anterior teeth;
7. Restore posterior teeth.

The first phase of treatment should result in a stabilized mouth with an adequate occlusion and basic restorations on healthy supporting tissues. The prognosis for each tooth needs to be reliable and teeth of dubious vitality should be root filled or, failing this, extracted. In any event, they should not be used as strategic teeth for a prosthesis if possible.

The posterior teeth should be restored with cores of good retention that can act to stabilize the teeth and the occlusion during the diagnostic period. Considerable difficulty will be experienced with dentinogenesis imperfecta, since the dentine may not be able to retain pins effectively. A combination of pins and dentine adhesive core material may work, but dentine fragility may make the teeth unrestorable.

Having established the basic foundation for advanced dentistry, accurate impressions should be taken and a precentric diagnostic mounting done (Ch. 12). A diagnostic waxing of the proposed occlusal scheme should be carried out using the wax added technique to establish the tooth contours required for restorations and pontics (or denture teeth). Where occlusal surfaces have been extensively lost, no occlusal reduction at the time of posterior preparations will be possible without loss of retention, and therefore the new restorations will have

to intrude into the freeway space. The amount of this intrusion will fix the occlusal plane level, and the incisor heights will be increased to match. Cusp height and slopes, and the new curve of Spee must match the proposed anterior guidance. It is wise to adopt the original shape of the curve of Spee.

The lower incisor tip is the starting point for determining the new anterior guidance. Its new position should be in line with the long axis of the tooth to maintain it in muscle balance. The height of the tip, determined from the new occlusal plane, in turn dictates the position of the cingulum centric stops on the upper incisors. The remainder of the incisor crowns can be shaped empirically at this stage to provide overbite and overjet consistent with the dental base relationship.

Clinically though, the upper incisor tip position will be determined by aesthetics, speech and muscle activity. Tooth length and width will need to match facial characteristics, but speech is the most important determinant. Use of the 'F' and 'S' sounds is important to relate the upper incisal edges to the lower lip.

The provisional restorations should be constructed to the diagnostic scheme, and care taken to adjust them correctly at the fitting stage.

Upon completion of the diagnostic waxing, this should be duplicated into stone, and remounted. The incisal table should be customized to the new guidance.

The next part of the diagnostic phase is to construct an occlusal splint which represents the increase in vertical dimension required by the new scheme and incorporates the predicted anterior guidance.

A lower splint, constructed from heat cured, hard acrylic resin, retained by cribs, is the most unobtrusive design. Initially, this is made from the pre-wax diagnostic mounting, with the articulator opened by the amount shown by the diagnostic waxing; the occlusal surface should be smooth.

On fitting, the splint is adjusted to provide even contact on closure on the retruded arc into centric relation. Since centric occlusion is being remodelled, it is now necessary to adopt centric relation as the reference position. The new centric occlusion position will be made coincident with centric relation at the new vertical dimension.

The patient should be manipulated onto the

retruded arc of closure (Ch. 12) and the splint marked with articulating paper at the retruded contact position. These markings should be indented to provide locating fossae for the new occlusal position.

The splint should be worn for about eight weeks, full time, to assess tolerance of the intrusion into the freeway space. After this has been successful, the preparations may be commenced.

The sequence should be:

1. Preparation of the twelve anterior teeth with the splint cut back to provide posterior support. Impressions and centric record;
2. Provisional restorations in accordance with the diagnostic waxing;
3. Trial cementation of the anterior crowns—speech, aesthetics and guidance checked and adjusted;
4. Posterior preparations with splint now discarded. Impressions and centric record;
5. Provisional restorations in accordance with the diagnostic waxing. Check for conformity of cusp slopes and height to the anterior guidance;
6. Trial cementation of posterior restorations;
7. Permanent cementation after review(s) and adjustment.

The centric record for both stages 1 and 4 is a centric relation record taken at the new vertical dimension. A recording splint is required whose thickness is equal to the height of the diagnostic splint and which locates accurately on the unprepared posteriors for stage 1 or the restored anteriors for stage 4. In this way, the mandible is guided into centric relation by the recording device and the preparation positions can be recorded by a ZOE wash (Fig. 19.4).

The new restorations are constructed and adjusted with CO ≡ CR, but there is some evidence that bony remodelling occurs to eventually re-establish a new centric relation position, posterior to new centric occlusion.

The maintenance of the final restorations requires periodic inspection by the dentist, but more important is the continued high standard of oral hygiene by the patient. The patient must be capable of preserving the restorations and be aware of the importance of their role (Figs 19.5 and 19.6).

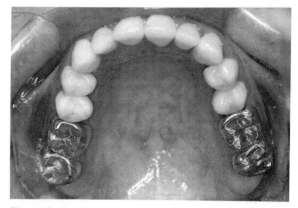

**Fig. 19.5** Reconstruction of the case shown in Figure 19.3. The anterior teeth are porcelain jacket crowns, the patient requested aesthetic occlusal surfaces for the metal–ceramic premolars, and the molars are full veneer crowns.

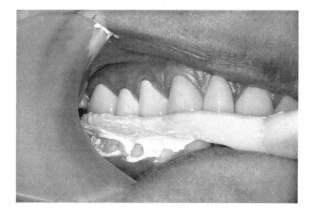

**Fig. 19.4** Occlusal registration splint in a case where the lower posterior teeth are being restored to an increased vertical dimension. The splint locates the mandible to the new vertical dimension on the retruded arc of closure, and the preparations are registered with a ZOE cement.

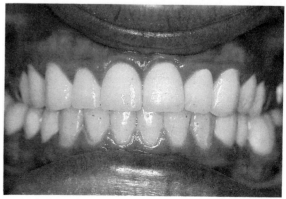

**Fig. 19.6** Centric occlusion of the case in Figure 19.5. The lower incisors were not restored.

## OVERDENTURES

These are technically less demanding and more cost effective in comparison with the provision of multiple crowns. They are the treatment of choice for the older patient with a number of missing teeth in addition to surface loss.

Essentially, the retention of healthy roots in the alveolus maintains the bony contours to provide support for dentures which are therefore likely to be more stable than conventional full dentures. The roots may be utilized to provide additional retention for the dentures.

The restorative options for the roots are, in order of increasing complexity:

1. Root filling (if a canal is present), reduction to gingival level and application of topical fluoride. Canal orifice sealed with amalgam;
2. Root filling and protective gold coping, retained by a cast post (Fig. 19.7);
3. As 2, but with gold coping increased in height to offer lateral resistance to denture movement;
4. As 2, but with precision retainer added to the coping to provide direct retention. Several systems exist for this purpose including the Eccentric (Rotherman) ring attachment or stud types, such as the Bona (Dalla Bona).

Where retention is not a problem, as in most upper dentures, the simplest option of tooth reduction without coping is very satisfactory. Cleaning of the root faces by the patient must be scrupulous, as the risk of caries is high.

Where insufficient alveolar ridge is present to provide good stability, particularly in lower dentures, then a shaped coping, or attachment, may be used. These have the disadvantage of subjecting the roots to lateral stress, which may accelerate periodontal breakdown. However, this may be a useful transition stage to the full denture.

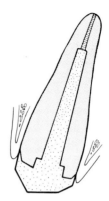

**Fig. 19.7** Diagram of a cast post and root cap for an overdenture. Note the long post and the root face bevel to increase stability.

The attachments also will be stressed during denture removal, and therefore the posts must be well made to resist cementation failure.

## CONCLUSIONS

There are immense variations between individual patients in their requirements, and in the ways in which treatment can be provided. This chapter has given a basic outline of the technical procedures involved, and their complexity, in providing multiple crowns, but the dentist is advised to approach these cases with caution.

Providing multiple crowns is not a single crown procedure repeated many times, and too often patients are asked to adapt to ill-conceived occlusal schemes with poorly constructed restorations.

To be successful, the work must be painstakingly planned and executed, and a high reliance placed on the patient's ability to maintain the restorations in a plaque and caries free state.

Prevention of surface loss is essential by recognizing that it is occurring and by providing the appropriate interceptive treatment.

# 20. Temporomandibular joint dysfunction

*P. H. Jacobsen*

Disorders of the temporomandibular joint (TMJ) may be categorized under the following headings:

- Acute muscle problems
- Inflammation of the joint
- Derangement of the joint
- Degenerative disease
- Extrinsic trauma
- Growth disorders

Conservative management is appropriate for the first and some aspects of the second and third, but the remainder tend to be managed by surgical techniques. This chapter will confine itself to discussion of conservative aspects of TMJ disorders.

## TEMPOROMANDIBULAR JOINT/MUSCLE DYSFUNCTION SYNDROME (TMJ/MDS)

This is essentially a musculo-skeletal disorder which is characterized by one or more of the following *in the absence of other oral pathology*.

- Mandibular movement problem; clicking, crepitus, incoordination
- Pain in the muscles or joints
- Restriction of movement

These may also be accompanied by parafunctional clenching or grinding — *bruxism*.

The disorder is characterized by a sequence of simple painless clicking followed by painful muscles and locking of the mandible, reaching a peak of pain which then declines. This decline may still be accompanied by clicking and crepitus in the joint. The period of the cycle may be several months or even years.

Surveys have indicated that 40% of the population may have the disorder during their lives. Classically, there is an episode in late teens which clears quickly, followed by a recurrence in middle age. Women are affected more than men and the principal symptoms are masticatory muscle pain or spasm, accompanied by clicking in the TMJs.

### Aetiology

The neuromuscular control of mandibular movement is extremely complex and was outlined in Chapter 7. There is a physiological requirement to stabilize the mandible during swallowing to provide a firm base from which the pharyngeal constrictor muscles can operate. The position of maximum stability is centric occlusion and whilst 'tooth apart swallows' are recognized, reaching centric occlusion 'smoothly' is a movement performed many times each day.

This movement is performed on a 'preferred arc of closure' which avoids any pre-centric interferences (Ch. 7). Being able to reach centric occlusion without touching interferences is partly learnt and partly reflex behaviour and, in the normal subject, is easily reproduced. Further, man has the capacity to adapt to and use many extremes of malocclusion quite successfully for functional purposes. Indeed, this adaptation can be quite rapid in the presence of, say a newly restored occlusal surface whose strangeness disappears after a few days.

However, several things may interfere with muscle and joint coordination which may have more lasting effects:

- Trauma, such as prolonged opening, wide yawning, or tough foods
- Pernicious habits such as nail biting, clenching or grinding

- 'Correction' of gross malocclusion by posture
- Extensive restorations or dentures of incorrect occlusal contour
- Independent oral pathology
- Emotional stress, anxiety, worry, major life event

The effects of trauma as an aetiological agent are very basic and can be understood clearly. Nail biting requires the mandible to be advanced to edge to edge incisal contact and maintained in that position for nibbling. The masticatory apparatus is not well suited to this function, and spasm may develop in the lateral pterygoid and masseter muscles.

Bruxism consists of continued parafunctional movements, which again cause the muscles to tire.

The moderate to gross Class II division I malocclusion causes problems in the achievement of a conventional oral seal and also, to compensate for the aesthetic problems of a chinless profile, subjects often posture forward continuously. This again fatigues the muscles.

The faulty occlusal surface induces an abnormal pattern of chewing, either because of avoidance, or because of awareness of a problem, and incoordination results. It is assumed that the adaptive capacity is exceeded in these cases.

Independent oral pathology is a major heading in the differential diagnosis of TMJ/MDS. The true syndrome occurs in the absence of such pathology, but sometimes the syndrome is induced by other disorders. These include carious teeth, pulpal conditions, apical pathology, split-roots — the list is very long. The aetiology is simply based on avoiding a painful or uncomfortable contact during function or parafunction.

The muscle and joint coordination is lost because a new pattern of movement is being attempted and joint clicking and muscle tenderness are the results.

Treatment to remove the pathology will usually induce the TMJ/MDS to resolve with no active occlusal therapy.

Emotional stress, anxiety or worry are considered to be major factors in the aetiology. These factors are recognized to be of importance in other conditions such as duodenal ulcer, low back pain and migraine, and TMJ/MDS falls into the group of psychosomatic pathology. Why some people get ulcers while others get facial pain is not clear. Psychological problems are complex and it is not for dental surgeons to play the amateur psychiatrist; however, some understanding is necessary.

The influence of the psychological factors would appear to be the interference with central functions. Again, the neural control of mastication is affected leading to incoordination. Other factors which may be stress related are clenching where parafunctional movement increases, and increase in the frequency of swallowing.

### Clinical features

The upshot of the complex aetiology is the greater or lesser development of the syndrome. The joint disturbance, which often occurs first, manifests itself as 'clicking', which may be painless. This disturbance must be clearly differentiated from dislocation of the joint which may occur on wide opening with the condyles slipping over a shallow articular eminence. This has been considered a feature of lax ligaments and 'hypermobility'.

The classic 'click' occurs on opening and/or closing with tooth separation of about 2–3 mm. This is caused by the articular disc becoming displaced from the head of the condyle and then 'catching up' either from a posterior or anterior position. The disc can become permanently displaced but this may be found in the absence of any symptoms at all. The click can be felt by palpation of the joints or heard via a stethoscope.

Failure of the relocation of the disc-condylar complex during opening can result in locking of the mandible at mid-opening. The disc is trapped anteriorly on or beyond the eminence. This again can be painless and patients may become used to relieving the problem themselves. However, once locking is accompanied by pain, the patient will seek treatment.

If treatment is not sought and the condition does not resolve, then progress of the disorder may continue with painful function, permanent displacement of the disc and eventually osteoarthritis. However, locking will usually have disappeared to be replaced by the pain from the joint in all functional positions.

The diagnosis of disc displacement is notoriously difficult to confirm since radiographs are often normal. To demonstrate the pathology, an arthrogram or computerized tomography (CT) scan is required.

The joint derangement may occur alone, but in patients seeking treatment it usually occurs in parallel with muscle pain and headache. Muscle pain, spasm or tenderness plus limitation of opening can occur without joint disturbance, but the reverse is unlikely.

The muscle pain can be initiated by a traumatic episode of chewing hard food or prolonged wide opening. It may be that the musculature has been already subjected to fatigue, possibly by clenching or by the neuro-muscular problems mentioned earlier. The superimposition of anxiety may reduce the pain threshold of the individual.

Bilateral palpation of each pair of masticatory muscles in turn is required to build up a picture of the severity of the disorder but subjectively this can be done by careful questioning. The extent of sleep loss, inability to chew and pain on opening will all contribute to an understanding of the extent of the problem; this in turn will give a guide to the possible success of treatment.

## Management

This is perhaps one of the most controversial areas of dentistry and the multitude of treatments that are used probably reflects the difficulty of accurate diagnosis and the low level of understanding of the pathology of the disorder.

The other complicating factor in the assessment of treatment methods is the self-limiting nature of the disease. There is definitely a peak of pain and dysfunction and then resolution, and much treatment is likely to be applied in the declining phase of the disease, thereby showing favourable results.

Broadly, conservative treatment may be categorized as follows:

1. Reassurance and explanation of the condition;
2. Basic physiotherapy;
3. Occlusal therapy;
4. Systemic therapy.

Of these, probably 3 and 4 are mutually exclusive, with practitioners having a strong preference for using one or the other. A balanced view would be that there is a place for all of these possibilities in the treatment of the condition, but the difficulty is to define the exact type of patient and syndrome which would benefit from which therapy.

There is some evidence to suggest that personality type or psychological morbidity have a bearing on the success of treatment. Some patients may be 'treatment seekers' and would not be satisfied with reassurance only. Others with a high psychological morbidity might be better treated with systemic antidepressants rather than local occlusal therapy.

There is a high level of placebo response reported in several studies and the confidence of the operator in the chosen therapy also influences the outcome.

### Reassurance and explanation

This is of fundamental importance, particularly in those patients who are in severe pain, who may have lost sleep and who find it difficult to eat. They need a simple explanation of the condition which will allay their fears that their condition is serious or even sinister.

An explanation based on the analogy of the pulled muscle or sprained ankle seems readily acceptable to most patients. The particular muscles involved can be demonstrated, and headache from the temporals or neckache from the sterno-mastoid or posterior belly of the digastric is easily explained. Clicking of the TMJs can also be compared to common clicking in other joints.

The relationship of the condition to anxiety or stress can be discussed, particularly if the patient admits to clenching or grinding during the day.

### Basic physiotherapy

This is to rest the affected muscles, ease spasm by the application of moist heat or cold (as in sports injury therapy) and the use of appliances, again to rest or support the affected parts.

Patients should be advised to avoid wide opening, to let their jaw hang loose to relax the muscles, and take a soft diet. An insulated hot water bottle is probably the most readily available way of applying heat to the muscles, though there are commercially available heat packs.

Having relieved muscle spasm, the jaws should be gently and steadily restored to normal function, either by positive exercise or by increasing the normality of the diet.

The exercises could be called neuromuscular retraining and one of the more popular is making symmetrical opening and closing movements from a central starting position. However, if these cause pain or fatigue they should be restricted. Indeed the use of exercises before the pain has been relieved by rest can be positively harmful.

The most common physiotherapeutic appliance is the occlusal splint which will be considered next.

### Occlusal therapy

This may consist of:

- Occlusal splint
- Occlusal equilibration
- Provision of restorations

**Occlusal splint**. The purpose of the splint is to rest the masticatory muscles and allow the musculature to place the mandible into whatever position is desired without being influenced by the teeth. The precision of centric occlusion requires the mandible to always reach this position for swallowing and this may not be the most comfortable position for the muscles with their neuro-muscular incoordination. The splint should introduce freedom of movement and also balance and stability to the mandible in its closed position.

A further function is to increase the muscle length which thereby reduces the power that can be generated by the muscles.

A large number of designs have been advanced and these include upper splints, lower splints, soft splints, hard splints, part occlusal coverage splints, total occlusal coverage splints, smooth splints, indented splints. The reader who would like to pursue this myriad of techniques is referred to the bibliography.

All designs seem to have moderate to good success rates and because of the particular history of TMJ/MDS, Solberg has suggested that the occlusal splint is 'the gold plated placebo'. The confidence of the operator in the splint could be very important in inducing a response by the patient.

The author has his own favourite occlusal splint, which works in his hands, and is described in detail below, together with his justification for using it.

The type and features are as follows:

1. Lower — this is less obstrusive than an upper and seems better tolerated;

2. Hard — accurate adjustment is possible together with exact stability on closure;
3. Smooth — allows freedom for the musculature to take the mandible to a range of stable positions;
4. Canine guided — posterior teeth are discluded and non-working interferences are eliminated.

Again, the explanation of the function of the splint to the patient is crucial to its success.

The splint is basically acrylic and can be made either in the laboratory as an articulated mounting of a pre-centric record, or from a vacuum formed plate which has cold-curing acrylic added at the chairside. The former is expensive of laboratory time and the latter is expensive of chairside time. The final features of each should be the same:

1. The base must be stable on the lower teeth, be retentive and not rock;
2. The supporting cusps of the upper premolars and molars should meet the splint with even contact on flat plateaux in any position from centric relation to centric occlusion and slightly anterior to that (long centric) (Fig. 20.1). This freedom of movement and evenness of contact should extend about 1 mm in each lateral direction. The patient should be able to slide smoothly on the splint by about 1 mm radius from centric occlusion;
3. There should be no incisal contact in long

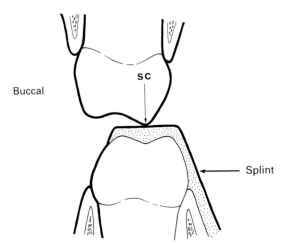

**Fig. 20.1** Transverse section of a splint in the molar region. The upper supporting cusp (SC) meets the splint on a flat plateau.

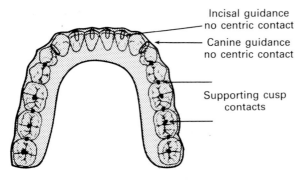

Incisal guidance
no centric contact

Canine guidance
no centric contact

Supporting cusp
contacts

**Fig. 20.2** Ideal occlusal contacts.

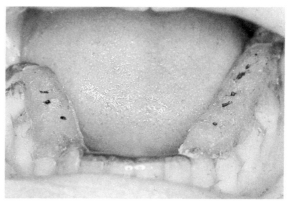

**Fig. 20.4** Articulating paper markings on a completed splint, showing the centric stop contacts. This splint is thicker than usual to disclude a deep anterior overbite.

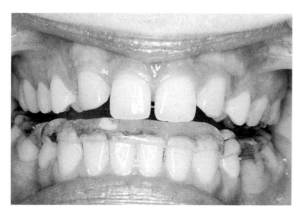

**Fig. 20.3** The anterior guide provides posterior disclusion on forward movement.

centric. This allows freedom in the arc of closure (Fig. 20.2);

4. Canine guidance should be incorporated by a raised plane anteriorly providing posterior disclusion;

5. Incisal guidance is provided in the same way, giving posterior disclusion in protrusion (Fig. 20.3).

The occlusal contacts should be checked carefully with articulating paper and shimstock (Fig. 20.4).

The splint should be worn full-time, particularly during eating and only removed for cleaning. It should be reviewed after one week and the occlusal contacts checked again, and then at four to six weekly intervals.

The resolution of the muscle pain is likely within two to three months, provided it is not severe and long standing. The superimposition of an internal derangement of the joint may require consideration

after the muscular pain has diminished (p. 194). Following relief of symptoms, a decision must be made as to whether it can be discarded or whether some occlusal treatment is required. Initially, the splint should be reduced to night wearing only for four weeks to judge response. If pain does not recur, then the splint can be left out altogether, followed again by review. The decision about long term therapy can then be made with confidence (Fig. 20.5).

Bruxism may also be treated by such a splint, though it should be heat cured for strength, and an upper one is usually more durable. Nights only wearing is quite successful as this is when most parafunction occurs. The bruxist should almost certainly continue nights only wearing for some considerable time.

***Occlusal equilibration***. This was discussed in Chapter 12. In relation to TMJ/MDS, some authorities recommend equilibration as a preventive measure as well as a treatment method. This author does not share these views and cautions against irreversible surface modification for a condition that is often self-resolving. Indeed, the occlusal disharmonies will have been present for some years prior to the commencement of the syndrome, and in many patients once the muscular pain has been resolved, they return to adapting to the disharmonies.

Certainly, equilibration should not be used as the primary treatment, since the musculature will be provoked by the periods of opening required for the

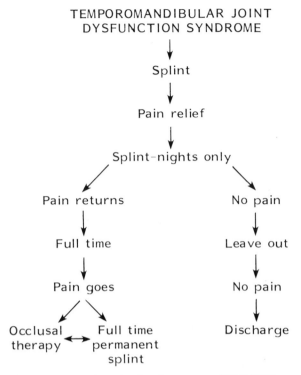

TEMPOROMANDIBULAR JOINT
DYSFUNCTION SYNDROME

↓

Splint

↓

Pain relief

↓

Splint-nights only

↙          ↘

Pain returns          No pain

↓                     ↓

Full time             Leave out

↓                     ↓

Pain goes             No pain

↙  ↘                  ↓

Occlusal  Full time   Discharge
therapy ↔ permanent
          splint

**Fig. 20.5** Flow chart showing the progress of TMJ/MDS with treatment.

therapy and CR is not likely to be reproducible with muscle pain and incoordination present.

If the pain is resolved by the use of the splint, then some workers consider this to be diagnostic of occlusal disharmonies being a primary aetiological agent. The complexity of the disorder, though, does not lend itself to such simple assumptions. A comparative study of equilibration versus feigned equilibration showed better resolution in the latter group.

Correction of major occlusal disharmonies is possibly of long term value. This would include orthodontic correction of instanding incisors, or the extraction of over-erupted wisdom teeth. There is some evidence to support the correction of a lateral deviation on closure into CO.

However, the presence of postero-anterior slides from CR to CO on closure is so common, that these really cannot be classed as aetiological agents in their own right. It may be that they become significant when the syndrome has developed, and their reversible elimination by a splint helps the syndrome

to resolve. But after this, they appear to return to their previous level of insignificance.

***Provision of restorations***. An incorrect occlusal surface can clearly initiate avoidance and then TMJ/MDS. In these cases the syndrome is secondary to the primary agent, the poor restoration, whose correction would be likely to eliminate the syndrome.

This approach can be used in mild cases, but in others the syndrome must be resolved first, before restorative therapy is commenced. This is again related to the likelihood of provoking the muscles by treatment and the difficulty in obtaining reproducible occlusal contact positions whilst the syndrome is present. The occlusal splint is without doubt appropriate here and is almost certain to succeed. Following this, re-restoration can be started.

Simple restoration replacement should be straightforward, but more extensive restorations can present difficulties. Alongside this, one can consider the problems of providing restorative therapy in general for resolved TMJ/MDS patients.

The dangers are that the provision of treatment could restart the syndrome by traumatizing the muscles, and also that the new restorations could restart it. The patient must also understand these dangers so that the operator is not held liable for the recurrence of the disorder.

Restorative therapy should be kept to the minimum possible and performed over short visits. An intra-oral prop should be used to give a firm platform on which to stabilize the muscles. If there is any sign of the syndrome during treatment, treatment should be suspended immediately. It may be necessary to reimplement the splint therapy and restabilize the condition.

*Systemic therapy*

Some systemic therapy may be used to accompany the occlusal splint. This could be analgesics (soluble aspirin is very effective) or muscle relaxants. The most common muscle relaxant for TMJ/MDS is diazepam but this should only be used for two or three days and then in very low doses of about 4 mg daily. The tranquilliser effect and the possibility of dependence is then very low.

The major use of systemic therapy is to counteract the central aetiological agents of stress and anxiety by prescribing antidepressants. The proponents of this approach argue that occlusal disharmonies may be present but they always have been, and that what has happened is a neuromuscular problem induced by interference with neural pathways. Tricyclic antidepressants are currently in vogue, and good success rates have been reported. However these are not substantially better than the rates for splint therapy.

The average dental surgeon, if he or she believes in this approach, should make the diagnosis and then refer the case to a medical practitioner for prescription. The side effects and dosage of anti-depressant therapy must be monitored and appropriate training is necessary to do this.

## INTERNAL DERANGEMENT

The articular disc may simply be out of phase with the condylar movement or may be permanently displaced. In addition, there may be derangement of the articular surfaces, either from trauma or from chronic inflammation. The simplest form of derangement is the click caused by the out of phase disc 'catching up' with the condyle, and if this is painless, no treatment is usually necessary. If the clicking is accompanied by muscle pain, then this should be stabilized first, and the result may be a painless click. Again, no active treatment for the residual click is necessary. The only problem is that the elastic fibres posterior to the disc, which bring it back from protrusion, can become stretched, leaving a prolapsed disc.

However, if the joint pain persists after splint therapy, together with limitation of opening and joint sounds, then further treatment is necessary. This is also true of locking, which can occur without clicking.

Further treatment must be done upon the basis of an accurate diagnosis and to do this, arthrograms of the TMJs are necessary. These will reveal whether the disc is displaced or whether there is arthritic or other changes in the joint. A spin-off from arthrography is that adhesions may be broken down

by the interference with the joint. This may be done intentionally with arthroscopy. Some success in curing locking has been reported.

Simple conservative therapy has some success in 'releasing' the displaced disc back to its normal position. This is done with a repositioning splint, which is very similar to the muscle stabilizing splint described earlier, but has positive tooth guiding planes for closure.

The path of closure is anterior to that normally employed, and the maximum contact position is forward also. Thus the condyles are advanced and pulled downwards in the fossae. The splint should be made from a wax record which reproduces the position of the mandible on closure just before the click occurs. The splint must be worn continuously and should not be used in the presence of muscle pain, which will be made worse by the abnormal forward posture.

Success rates for repositioning splint therapy are variable and this type of therapy should be reserved for those cases which have remained insoluble from the muscle stabilization splint.

The internal derangements resulting from trauma or osteoarthritic change require surgical management.

## CONCLUSIONS

The condition remains a controversial area because of the difficulties of defining and diagnosing the syndrome and the large number of treatments, including placebo, which have reasonable success rates.

Simple, reversible, non-invasive therapies are recommended as the first option with the more difficult procedures and systemic drug therapy held in reserve for those who do not respond to the first approach.

There is clearly a small group of patients who show little response to all forms of treatment, and who eventually get better by themselves.

# 21. Management of failures

*P. H. Jacobsen*

We all have failures; but it is essential to learn from them and not make the same mistake again. This book has tried to give a practical, commonsense approach to many aspects of conservative dentistry, and to follow its advice, the authors believe, would reduce the incidence of failures.

The two major reasons for failure are treatment planning errors and technical errors.

The treatment plan must be tailored to fit the patient and be based on an accurate diagnosis of the pathologies present (Ch. 4). It must also fit the dentist's skills and facilities. For instance, a treatment plan based on the skills and experience of a hospital specialist and supporting team is likely to be quite beyond the reach of the average general practitioner.

Poor treatment planning, then, is a major problem, often compounded by technical errors. Simple plans, made up of easy stages are always best, no matter how skilled the operator. Unreasonable demands on technical expertise that does not exist, and patient motivation and awareness that is half-hearted are recipes for disaster.

Thankfully, a lot of less-than-perfect dentistry requires no treatment, other than regular observation. The criteria to be applied before embarking on wholesale re-restoration are:

- Is there any active pathology in the area of the problem?
- Are there any symptoms?
- Is there an aesthetic problem that disturbs the patient?
- Is there a functional problem?

If the answer is 'yes' to any of these, then action is required; but there are many examples of imperfection, where nothing should be done.

## EXAMPLES FOR MASTERLY INACTIVITY

### The ditched, corroded amalgam restoration

This type of restoration should not be replaced unless there is evidence of recurrent caries, either clinically or radiographically, or there are symptoms of microleakage (Fig. 3.3).

### The under- or over-filled root canal

This should not be interfered with unless there are clinical or radiographic signs of an enlarging apical area, or symptoms. If the decision is made to interfere, then the operator should be certain that they can do better. Is the canal apical to the short filling obstructed, for example?

## INTRACORONAL RESTORATIONS

### 'Cracked tooth syndrome'

This condition can cause considerable difficulty in diagnosis. It involves a hairline, vertical fracture extending from the base of a large cavity, either to the root furcation, or down the root as well. The patient will complain of vague symptoms, perhaps mainly on biting, which are often poorly localized. Radiographs will usually show no abnormality. If infection supervenes, then the affected tooth may be tender, but again there are usually no radiographic signs.

The affected tooth will usually have a large MOD amalgam present, again possibly with no apparent defects. Removal of the amalgam will reveal a deep occlusal floor and a flat plastic should be gently turned within the cavity to attempt to open the buccal wall from the lingual. A crack in the floor may then be revealed.

The prognosis for the tooth is poor, though symptoms may be relieved by placing an acid-etched composite restoration. The cusps will be held together, thus preventing the flexure which stimulates the periodontium. However, the fracture line is vulnerable to infection, which may occur at any time.

**Dentine pins**

Pins in the periodontal ligament or pulp are a complication which can be unavoidable, due to the blind nature of their insertion. The misplacement of the pinhole should be diagnosed as soon as it has been drilled; either because the resistance to cutting was suddenly lost, or because blood appeared in the hole.

The hole should not be used, but filled with calcium hydroxide. However, if a pin has been inadvertently placed in such a hole, then pulpal or periodontal infection can occur. Treatment of the pulpal infection might require root canal therapy, whilst the periodontal infection may require raising a flap, cutting the excess pin away and smoothing it flush with the root.

If the pin is superficial, then a crown preparation could cover it as a method of sealing. If the pin is inaccessible, then extraction could be the only solution.

Beware of interpreting the two dimensional radiograph incorrectly. A correctly placed pin may be superimposed on the pulp shadow (Fig. 21.1).

## POST CROWNS

These are particularly vulnerable to operator error during preparation. The root morphology is unknown and unseen, and it is easy to be misled by an apparently large root face which tapers dramatically in the alveolus.

The side of the post hole may be perforated during preparation, or the root may be weakened leading to vertical fracture during preparation, cementation or later function. Posts may fracture in the canal.

**Lateral perforation**

Large, parallel sided posts are prone to this complication and particular teeth are also vulnerable. The upper lateral incisor being small and angulated

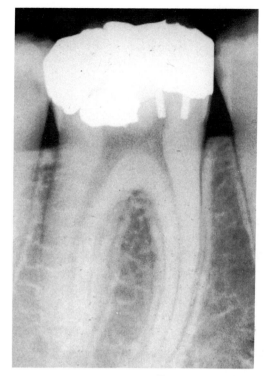

**Fig. 21.1** Periapical radiograph of 6̄| with a pin apparently in the pulp. It is, in fact, buccal and correctly placed.

distally and palatally is a particular trap, as are roots with mesial and distal concavities (p. 199).

Teeth that can be either two-rooted or single rooted, such as upper premolars, also give rise to problems, simply because the root morphology is unseen.

Perhaps the best advice is to avoid posts in teeth which are known to be variable in morphology, and construct pinned cores instead (Ch. 10).

The differential diagnosis for a post crowned tooth which is giving problems must always include the possibility of a perforation, and a second radiographic view can be helpful (Fig. 21.2). This will also show the position of the perforation as labial or palatal by parallax.

The management of the lateral perforation depends upon its site and size, and the restorability and prognosis of the tooth as a whole. A carious, short rooted tooth is better extracted, rather than embarking upon difficult treatment. Also, if a perforation can be positively diagnosed as palatally placed, then the tooth should be extracted.

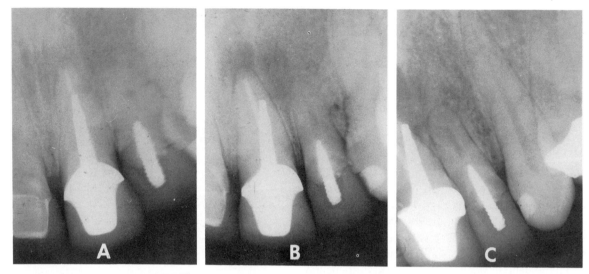

**Fig. 21.2** Periapical radiographs of the |12 region. **A**, suggests that the post is in the correct line of the canal; **B**, taken to show the |2, reveals the post off-line; **C**, taken for the |3, reveals a palatal perforation of |1. Unfortunately, the original diagnosis had been made using A only, and the patient had been treated for TMJ dysfunction. The central incisor was later extracted.

Having decided upon trying to save the tooth, the first decision is whether to remove the offending post, or leave it in situ. A small rooted tooth may not survive the stress involved in withdrawing a post, and a threaded post can stress the root excessively on being unscrewed.

If the post can be removed (or if the perforation has been observed at preparation), then the post hole should be re-established in the correct line (Fig. 21.3), an impression taken and the new post fitted at the time of surgical exposure of the perforation.

The perforation should be isolated so that cement does not enter the bone, and the post cemented with polycarboxylate cement. An acrylic provisional crown should be placed as well. The perforation should be cleaned and retention provided around it

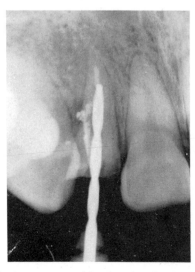

**Fig. 21.3** A post crown with a lateral perforation has been removed, and the canal re-established in the correct line.

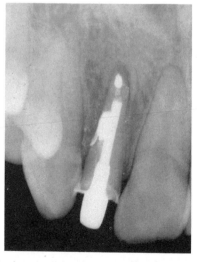

**Fig. 21.4** A new post was constructed and cemented at apical surgery. The perforation has been repaired with amalgam, and a retrograde root filling placed.

by a small round bur. Amalgam should then be placed to seal the perforation (Fig 21.4). This procedure may be complicated by the wedge shaped nature of the perforation, which may be long in the long axis of the tooth and whose walls can be very thin.

If the original post cannot be removed, then surgical repair may be attempted by removing the post material that is outside the root profile, and cutting a channel around its end. This is then filled with amalgam.

A small perforation, noticed at the time of preparation, may be packed with calcium hydroxide from within the canal, the post made in the correct line, cemented as usual, and periodically reviewed radiographically.

## Two cautionary tales

### A diagnostic disaster 1

The case illustrated in Figure 21.5 had a post crown constructed on the upper left lateral incisor some eight years previously. The tooth had given problems subsequently, and an apicectomy was performed. This did not resolve the problem and the patient, having moved home, consulted a new practitioner.

The practitioner said that the previous apicectomy had failed, and the operation should be repeated. He provided the root seal shown in Figure 21.5A.

The tooth still gave trouble, and a further house move brought the patient yet another adviser. The hospital practitioner who saw her advised that the second apicectomy had failed, and that the operation

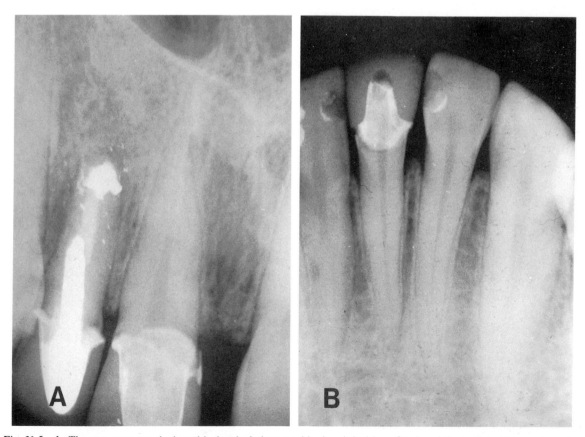

**Fig. 21.5  A**, The post crown on the lateral incisor had given trouble since it had been fitted, and the tooth had been apicected twice previously, with no benefit. There is no apical pathology present on the crowned 1|; **B**, The lower central incisor had a badly fitting crown, but no apical pathology. The practitioner prescribed a further apicectomy for 2|, and because of negative pulp tests on 1| and |1, apicectomies were prescribed for these as well.

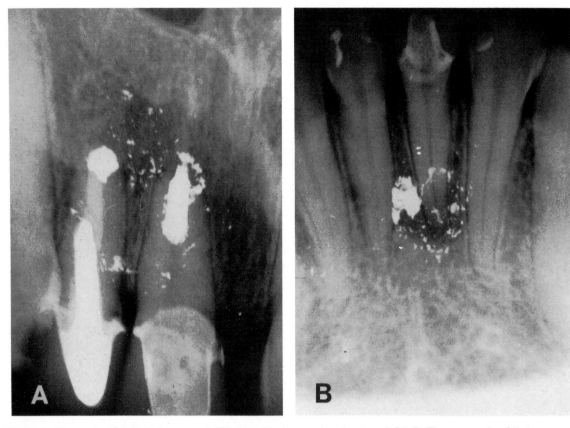

**Fig. 21.6** The results of the apical surgery. **A**, The lateral incisor continued to be painful; **B**, The operator has failed to identify the apex of ⌐T and has deposited amalgam in bone. The tooth was subsequently found to be vital.

should be repeated. He also tested the vitality of the crowned central incisor and the crowned lower incisor (Fig. 21.5B) with ice and concluded that they were non-vital. (Porcelain is a good insulator!) He advised that both these teeth should be apicected also, in spite of the *absence of any apical pathology*.

After a nine month wait, the three apicectomies were done by a further practitioner, as a day case. He provided the surgical results shown in Figure 21.6.

The upper lateral still did not recover, and the patient was seen by the author. Surgical investigation of the strong possibility of a lateral perforation by the off-line post was done, a perforation found and repaired, and the tooth settled. The lower incisor turned out to be vital, was root filled and post crowned, and the large mass of misplaced amalgam left under review.

The patient pressed a successful claim for damages, and all teeth were still present and symptomless four years later.

*A diagnostic disaster 2*

The upper second premolar illustrated in Figure 21.7 had given trouble since the post crown had been fitted. Acute inflammation developed such that the whole quadrant was painful with all the teeth being tender.

The patient attended a Sunday morning emergency service and for some reason, the dentist diagnosed acute apical infection of the two perfectly sound incisors of the upper left side. These were 'opened to drain' and the patient attended hospital the next day.

The vital pulps, still present in the incisors, were extirpated and the teeth root filled later. The patient elected to have the perforated premolar extracted. No legal action resulted.

This case illustrates firstly, the danger of making posts on roots with unseen concavities, and secondly, the need to have the fullest information available before a committed diagnosis is made.

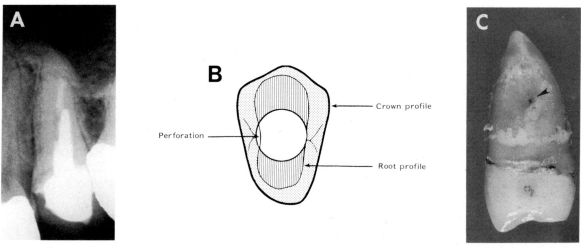

**Fig. 21.7** **A,** The radiograph shows the post in ⌊5 to be slightly off line, but not dramatically so. However, the root profile of single rooted upper premolars tends to have concavities (**B**), which cannot be seen. The large crown profile gives a false sense of security, but a perforation has occurred (**C,** arrowed).

In the face of seven tender teeth in a quadrant and no radiographs, the prescription of analgesics and antibiotics is a safer course of action.

### Vertical fracture

Complete vertical fracture is often the consequence of a blow or jar to a post crown which knocks it out. Short, or ill fitting, posts are particularly vulnerable. Diagnosis may not be obvious, but root integrity must be checked before recementing the crown. A small flat plastic instrument should be inserted into the post hole, and turned gently to open any fracture line (Fig 21.8). Excessive force is not necessary and should be avoided. In the event of a vertical fracture, the tooth cannot be saved.

Incomplete fracture is very difficult to diagnose. It is an occasional finding during apical surgery, and all roots with posts should be inspected carefully at the time of surgery.

The crack, or cracks, may have been caused by overzealous preparation with large twist drills, or by a later blow. They can remain stable for some time, but in some cases tissue fluid leaks through and initiates corrosion, either of the post or of a metallic root filling.

The corrosion products open the fracture line, infection supervenes, and the tooth gives symptoms. The tooth cannot be saved, but diagnosis may not be made until surgery is attempted, at which time a stained root is revealed (Fig 21.9).

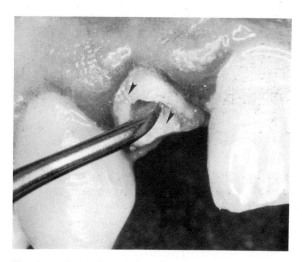

**Fig. 21.8** Check for root fracture when a post crown has been lost. The flat plastic is twisted gently in the canal and the fracture (arrowed) has opened.

Vertical fractures may also be caused by tapered, threaded posts upon insertion. These are dangerous and should not be used.

### Fractured post

This is a particular complication of cast posts or small posts of all types. A blow, or a jar during eating, shears the post at a casting defect. The root should be

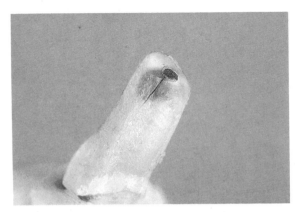

**Fig. 21.9** A partly fractured root which has allowed tissue fluid to reach the metal post, and corrosion has resulted. This was found at apicectomy and the tooth was later extracted.

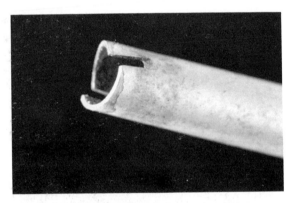

**Fig. 21.10** A Masserann trepan. The cutting tube removes cement or dentine from around the object in the canal, which is thereby released.

checked for vertical fracture, and if intact, removal of the fragment performed.

A special kit (Masserann, Micro-Mega) is recommended (Fig 21.10). This is a series of cutting tubes (trepans) which are designed to cut an annulus around the fragment, thus releasing it. The tooth can then be re-restored.

## CROWN AND BRIDGEWORK

### Cementation failure

This can be very difficult to diagnose, since it may be partial, with the crown apparently still secure. The patient may report vague symptoms that will relate initially to dentine stimulation by microleakage and then to carious attack. These symptoms may not be specific to one tooth, and in a multiple unit restoration, this can be preplexing.

Radiographs will not reveal anything at the early stage, unless there is a deficient crown margin. Applying displacing pressure to the restoration may reveal looseness or tell-tale bubbles at the cervical margin. This can be helpful in single crowns or on one side of a pontic, but multiple retainers may be supporting the failed one. Unfortunately, the diagnosis can only be made with confidence when the crown is fully unseated, by which time caries could have destroyed most of the preparation (Fig. 21.11).

All this points to choosing luting agents of the highest possible resistance to dissolution and fitting bridges with the best possible marginal adaptation and retention.

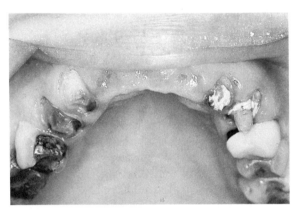

**Fig. 21.11** The preparations found under a failed bridge replacing 21|1 from 3|23 which had been fitted eighteen months previously. Cementation failure coupled with poor retention has lead to considerable recurrent caries and pulpal involvement.

Once cementation failure has been diagnosed on a bridge, the whole restoration must be removed without damage (p. 203), the integrity of the abutments checked and the bridge recemented if the abutments are satisfactory.

### Recurrent caries

This is potentially serious, since once the preparation dentine is reached, caries can spread rapidly. It will be revealed at routine maintenance visits, either by clinical or radiographic observation. Provided it is limited to the immediate area of the margin, the caries can be removed and the area restored with glass ionomer cement. A more extensive zone of caries, and particularly any that runs some way out of sight under a retainer, will necessitate the removal of the crown.

## Incorrect occlusion

This may give the patient the feeling that the teeth do not meet evenly, or worse, induce TMJ dysfunction.

The occlusion should be examined first with articulating paper and shimstock, as described in Chapter 12. If the discrepancies are seen clearly and are not large, simple equilibration can be successful. Where there is any doubt about the errors, a diagnostic pre-centric mounting should be done to permit clear examination of the occlusal contacts. A trial equilibration can be carried out on the articulation, and, if successful, repeated on the patient. If the discrepancies are too large, then the bridge will require remaking (p. 203).

If the bridge appears to have induced TMJ dysfunction, then this condition must be stabilized first and under no circumstances should there be any irreversible adjustments made to the bridge. It is possible that the dysfunction was coincidental with the bridge fitting, and not actually caused by it. Once the dysfunction has been resolved (Ch. 20), a detailed examination of the bridge can be made. Figure 21.12

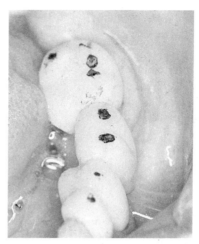

Fig. 21.13 The new bridge shows even contact in group function. The patient requested aesthetic crowns throughout.

shows a bridge with uneven occlusion, that induced TMJ/MDS. The condition was stabilized with a splint and then the bridge was remade (Fig. 21.13).

## Fractured ceramic

Small areas may be repaired using a proprietary silane coupling agent and a composite resin. More extensive loss will require that the restoration be remade (Fig. 21.14).

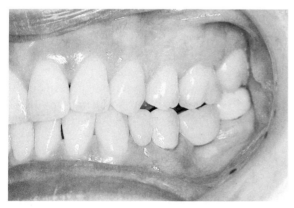

Fig. 21.12 This bridge in the lower left quadrant had poor occlusal contact and had induced TMJ dysfunction syndrome. The syndrome was stabilized by means of a splint, and when the patient was pain free, the bridge was remade.

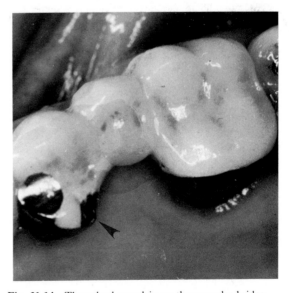

Fig. 21.14 The palatal porcelain on the premolar bridge retainer has fractured because it was too thin. The cusp should have been reduced to accommodate metal and porcelain, or better still, replaced by metal only.

## Management of the failed bridge

A bridge may be a candidate for replacement if:

- There is recurrent caries
- There is cementation failure
- One or more abutments show active pulpal or apical pathology
- One or more retainers show bad marginal adaptation
- The aesthetics are unacceptable
- The function is unacceptable

Limited recurrent caries might be amenable to local excavation and restoration, and a single pulpally involved tooth in an otherwise acceptable bridge, could be root filled through the retainer.

In other cases, particularly where several of the replacement criteria are fulfilled, removal of the bridge is the only satisfactory solution. Because the basic condition of the abutments is hidden by the retainers, the patient must be clearly informed that no guarantees can be given about the eventual re-restoration. They must understand that if the abutment teeth prove to be unsatisfactory, a partial denture could be the end result.

The sequence for management is:

1. Preoperative diagnostic mounting;
2. Provisional replacement constructed, usually a partial denture;
3. Remove the bridge;
4. Section bridge into individual retainers for use as provisional crowns; fit denture;
5. Inspect and assess each abutment tooth — vitality, restorability, prognosis;
6. Stabilize abutment teeth as appropriate — e.g. RCT, pinned cores;
7. Plan new bridge, (or alternative replacement);
8. Construct new bridge.

Perhaps the most difficult stage is the removal of the old bridge. Since it may be desirable to use the retainers as individual provisional crowns, removal should create the least damage possible. There is, of course, the very real danger of damaging the abutment teeth as well.

Gentle prising, by placing a Mitchell's trimmer or chisel at each retainer margin in turn, should be tried first. Then, if no movement results, mechanical shock can be applied to each retainer in an attempt to break the lute seal. Ultrasonic scalers can be successful, but the hammer blows of proprietary crown removers are more common. These are particularly unpleasant for the patient, and can fracture teeth underneath the bridge if not used with extreme care. Again, if no movement is seen after a few minutes the last resort is to cut each retainer with the air turbine. This technique, whilst destroying the bridge, at least means that the abutments escape with minimal damage.

A vertical cut should be made on the buccal aspect of each retainer, though the metal/ceramic only, using the appearance of the luting agent as a guide to depth. Special burs are available to do this. Care should be taken not to cut dentine, since this leaves grooves which may dictate an unfavourable path of insertion for the new bridge. A cut across the occlusal surface may also be necessary for the retainer to be released.

To construct the provisional restorations, temporary crown forms may be used, or alternatively, the preoperative mounting can be used as the template for resin-based provisional crowns (Fig. 21.15).

## THE OBSESSIVE PATIENT

This is a failure, or series of failures waiting to happen. Feinmann and Harris have coined the term 'oral dysaesthesia' for patients who have an unnatural concern about their dentitions.

Dentists and plastic surgeons are very vulnerable to the demands of perfection seeking individuals, and in dentistry, whilst sometimes reasons for treatment can be found, no organic disorder will usually be found to underlie the request for treatment. (This is the third time this warning has been written in this book — we think it bears repeating.)

Such patients may complain about the aesthetics of their teeth or the arrangement of their 'bite'. In the writer's experience, many are women in their thirties, with apparently stable family backgrounds.

Other patients, particularly in the older age groups, complain of pain for which no organic pathology can be found. Some also give impossible pathologies as their diagnosis, e.g. a patient believed that microleakage around a crown lead to air entering the nervous system and causing paralysis of the left side at night!

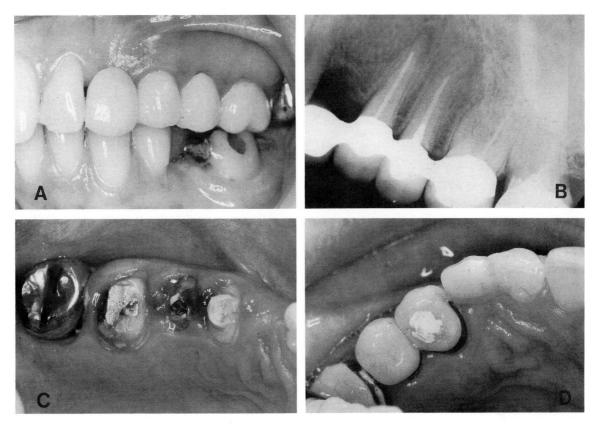

**Fig. 21.15**  **A**, This bridge replacing |3 is cantilevered from |456, which is probably one retainer too many; **B**, The radiograph shows that the premolar crowns have poor margins and short root fillings. There is an apical area on the |4, and a second root which has not been filled. The buccal root canals of |6 have not been filled; **C**, The underlying teeth showing recurrent caries, and inadequate preparations on the premolars; **D**, The bridge has been sectioned into individual provisional crowns to allow the root canal therapy to be redone, and a denture tooth has been acid-etched to the |2. Following the root therapy, the bridge was remade from |45, with the |6 being restored with an individual crown.

The dentist can easily be tempted by the history to undertake replacement of the dubious amalgam, provide crowns or even extract perfectly healthy teeth. Unless a pathological process is diagnosed, *no operative treatment* should be performed. This will be doomed to failure, and the patient will continue to demand more and more until the dentist calls a halt. The patient will then leave in a distressed state.

Recognition of the problem is the key to avoiding it. One should beware of the patient who asks numerous technical questions, offers a history of unsatisfactory care elsewhere or who is over-bearingly demanding about the standards of care required.

## MEDICO-LEGAL ASPECTS OF FAILURES

Every patient with a failed restoration is a potential litigant, but fortunately the vast majority of patients are loyal to their professional advisers. By discussing possible problems as they are foreseen during treatment, the patient is taken into the dentist's confidence and, if the worst happens, the patient is forewarned. The patient may then sympathize with the dentist. The ability of the dentist to communicate effectively is a major factor in avoiding litigation.

When discussing failures with the patient, it is important to put the problem in the context of the general difficulty of the technical aspects of dentistry. Explanations about the variation in tooth form, technique sensitive materials and so on, often gain the patient's sympathy and understanding.

However, this is not to suggest that deceiving the patient is appropriate. It is very necessary to explain exactly what is wrong and what needs to be done to put it right, without apportioning blame. If the patient continues to express dissatisfaction with previous care, it is best to be non-committal and supportive of the previous dentist if at all possible.

The courts do not expect every dentist to have specialist skills and to be successful in every case. They require that the treatment provided is appropriate to the dentist's training and experience, and has been delivered in a careful manner.

# Bibliography

## SECTION 1
## THE PATIENT

### Medical history

British Dental Association 1987 Guide to bloodborne viruses and the control of cross-infection in dentistry. British Dental Association, London

Cawson R A 1984 Essentials of dental surgery. 4th edn. Churchill Livingstone, Edinburgh

Cawson R A 1985 Use of antibiotics in dentistry. In: Rowe A H R (ed.) Companion to dental studies. Blackwell, Oxford

DHSS 1986 Guidelines for surgeons, anaesthetists and dentists in dealing with HTLV III. HMSO, London

Farthing C F, Brown S E, Staughton R C D, Cream J J, Michelmann M 1986 A colour atlas of AIDS. Wolfe, London

Franks A S T, Hedegard B 1973 Geriatric dentistry. Blackwell, Oxford

McGowan D A 1982 Endodontics and infective endocarditis. International Endodontic Journal 158: 127–151

Porter S R, Scully C, Cawson R A 1987 AIDS: update and guidelines for general dental practice. Dental Update 14: 336–339

### Periodontology

Greene J C, Vermillion J R 1964 The simplified oral hygiene index. Journal of the American Dental Association 68: 7–10

Lindhe J 1983 Textbook of clinical periodontology. Munksgaard, Copenhagen

### Radiography

Browne R M, Edmundson H D, Rout P G J 1983 A radiographic atlas of diseases of the teeth and jaws. Wiley, New York

Mason R 1983 A guide to dental radiography. 2nd edn. Wright, Bristol

### Anaesthesia, analgesia and sedation

Edmunds D H, Rosen M 1977 Sedation for conservative dentistry. Journal of Dentistry 5: 245–251

Kaufmann L, Rood J P, Sowray J H 1986 Sedation and general anaesthesia. In: Rowe A H R (ed.) Companion to dental studies. Blackwell, Oxford

Roberts D, Sowray J H 1979 Local analgesia in dentistry. 2nd edn. Wright, Bristol

Roberts G J 1979 Relative analgesia — an introduction. Dental Update 6: 271–284

### Trauma

Andreasson J O 1972 Traumatic injuries of the teeth. Munksgaard, Copenhagen

## SECTION 2
## THE RESTORATION AND ITS ENVIRONMENT

### Oral biology and pathology

Fearnhead R W, Suga S 1984 Tooth enamel IV. Elsevier, Amsterdam

Kidd E A M, Joyston-Bechel S 1987 Essentials of dental caries. Wright, Bristol

McKay G S 1976 The histology and microbiology of acute occlusal dentine lesions in human permanent molar teeth. Archives of Oral Biology 21: 51–58

Mjor I A, Fejerskov O 1986 Human embryology and histology. Munksgaard, Copenhagen

Osborn J W 1973 Variation in structure and development of enamel. Oral Science Reviews 3: 8–83

Silverstone L M 1973 Structure of carious enamel including the early enamel lesion. Oral Science Reviews 3: 100–160

Thylstrup A, Fejerskov O 1986 Textbook of cariology. Munksgaard, Copenhagen

### Occlusion

Alexander P C 1965 The periodontium and the canine function theory. Journal of Prosthetic Dentistry 18: 571–577

Bennett N G 1908 A contribution to the study of the movement of the mandible. Transactions of the Royal Society of Medicine 1: 77–84

Beyron H L 1969 Optimal occlusion. Dental Clinics of North America, 13: 537–542

Celenza F V 1973 The centric position: replacement and character. Journal of Prosthetic Dentistry 30: 591–595

D'Amico A 1961 Functional occlusion of the natural teeth of man. Journal of Prosthetic Dentistry 11: 899–915

Jent T, Lundquist S, Hedegard B 1982 Group function or canine protection. Journal of Prosthetic Dentistry 18: 719–720

Lauritzen A G, Bodner G H 1961 Variations in location of arbitrary and true hinge axis points. Journal of Prosthetic Dentistry 11: 224–229

Linde J, Nyman S 1977 The role of occlusion in periodontal disease and the biologic rationale for splinting in the treatment of periodontitis. Oral Sciences Review 10: 11–17

Posselt U 1957 Movement areas of the mandible. Journal of Prosthetic Dentistry 7: 375–379

Ramfjord S, Ash M M 1983 Occlusion. 3rd edn. Saunders, Philadelphia

Schuyler S H 1969 Freedom in centric. Dental Clinics of North America 13: 681–685

## Restorative materials

Beech D R 1973 Improvement in the adhesion of polyacrylate cements to human dentine. British Dental Journal 135: 442–445

Causton B E 1984 Improved bonding of composite restoratives to dentine. British Dental Journal 156: 93–95

Craig R J 1988 Restorative dental materials. Mosby, St Louis

Fusayama T 1979 Non-pressure adhesion of a new adhesive restorative resin. Journal of Dental Research 58: 1364–1370

Jacobsen P H 1984 The restoration of Class II cavities by polymeric materials. Journal of Dentistry 12: 47–52

Jacobsen P H 1986 Extension of the working time of light activated composite materials. British Dental Journal 160: 162–165

Jacobsen P H 1987 Biological and clinical testing of materials. Journal of Dentistry 15: 266–268

Jacobsen P H 1988 Design and analysis of clinical trials. Journal of Dentistry 16: 215–218

Munksgaard E C, Asmussen E 1984 Bond strength between dentine and restorative resins mediated by mixtures of HEMA and glutaraldehyde. Journal of Dental Research 63: 1087–1089

Osborne J et al 1978 Clinical performance and physical properties of twelve amalgam alloys. Journal of Dental Research 57: 963–988

Sarkar N F 1978 Creep, corrosion and marginal fracture of dental amalgams. Journal of Oral Rehabilitation 5: 413–423

Vanherle G, Smith D C 1985 (eds) Posterior composite materials. 3M, St. Paul

Wilson A D, McLean J W 1988 Glass ionomer cements. Quintessence, Chicago

## SECTION 3
## CLINICAL AND TECHNICAL PROCEDURES

### Intracoronal restorations

Brannstrom M, Isaacson G, Johnson G 1976 Effect of calcium hydroxide and fluorides on human dentine. Acta Odontologica Scandinavia 34: 59–66

Cohen S, Burns R C 1987 Pathways to the pulp. 4th edn. Mosby, St Louis

Elderton R D 1971 A modern approach to the use of rubber dam. Dental Practitioner and Dental Record 21: 187–191, 226–230, 267–273

Jacobsen P H, Robinson P B 1981 Basic techniques and materials for conservative dentistry, 3: Restoration of the broken down posterior tooth. Journal of Dentistry 9: 101–108

Nicholls E N 1984 Endodontics. 3rd edn. Wright, Guildford

Oligushi K, Fusayama T 1975 Electron microscope structure of the two layers of carious dentine. Journal of Dental Research 54: 1019–1026

Outhwaite W C, Garman T A, Pashley D H 1979 Pins v. slot retention in extensive amalgam restorations. Journal of Prosthetic Dentistry 41: 396–400

Rodda J C 1972 Modern class II amalgam cavity preparation. New Zealand Dental Journal 68: 132–136

Wein F S 1982 Endodontic therapy. 3rd edn. Mosby, St Louis

## Extracoronal restorations

Cruickshanks-Boyd D W 1981 Alternatives to gold. 2. Porcelain bonding alloys. Dental Update 8: 111–119

Friedman J 1973 The technical aspects of electro-surgery. Oral Surgery 36: 177–187

Harty F J, Leggett L J 1972 Post crown technique using a nickel–cobalt–chromium post. British Dental Journal 132: 394–397

Henry P, Bower R 1977 Post and core systems in crown and bridge. Australian Dental Journal 22: 46–52

Howard W S, Newman S M, Nunez L J 1980 Castability of low gold content alloys. Journal of Dental Research 59: 824–830

Kelly J R, Rose T C 1983 Non-precious alloys for use in fixed prosthodontics. A literature review. Journal of Prosthetic Dentistry 49: 363–370

McCabe J F, Wilson H J 1978 Addition curing silicone rubber impression materials. British Dental Journal 145: 17–20

McLean J W, Sced I 1976 The bonded alumina crown 1. The bonding of platinum to aluminous dental porcelain using tin oxide coatings. Australian Dental Journal 21: 119–127

## Adhesive techniques

Garber D, Goldstein R, Feinman R 1988 Porcelain laminate veneers. Quintessence, Chicago

Simonsen R, Thompson V, Barrack G 1983 Etched cast restorations. Clinical and laboratory techniques. Quintessence, Chicago

Tay W M 1986 Classification and assessment of composite retained bridges. Restorative Dentistry 2: 15–18

Tay W M 1988 Resin bonded bridges. 1. Materials and methods. Dental Update 15: 10–14

## Bridgework

Jacobsen P H 1981 The missing incisor. 2. Fixed bridgework. Dental Update 9: 45–49

Nyman S, Ericsson I 1982 Capacity of reduced periodontal

tissues to support fixed bridgework. Journal of Clinical Periodontology 9: 409–412

Prieskel H W 1984 Precision attachments in prosthodontics. Application of intracoronal and extracoronal attachments. Quintessence, Chicago

Shillingburg H T, Hobo S, Whitsett L D 1981 Fundamentals of fixed prosthodontics. 2nd edn. Quintessence, Chicago

# SECTION 4
# PROBLEMS

## Temporomandibular joint dysfunction

Feinmann C, Harris M 1984 Psychogenic facial pain. British Dental Journal 156: 165–170, 205–209

Greene C S, Laskin D M 1972 Splint therapy for myofacial pain dysfunction syndrome: a comparative study. Journal of the American Dental Association 84: 624–628

Solberg W K 1986 Temporomandibular disorders. British Dental Association, London

## Failures

Jacobsen P H 1982 and 1983 Failures in conservative dentistry.
1. Intracoronal restorations. Dental Update 9: 421–427
2. Endodontics. Dental Update 9: 477–484
3. Apical surgery. Dental Update 9: 525–534
4. Crowns. Dental Update 10: 9–16
5. Bridgework. Dental Update 10: 73–81

# Index